THE GLADIATOR DIET

THE GLADIATOR DIET

Larrian Gillespie

Healthy Life
publications

Visit our website at
http://GLADIATORDIET.COM

Healthy Life Publications Inc.
264 S. La Cienega Blvd., PMB #1233
Beverly Hills, Calif. 90211
1-800-554-3335
1-310-471-2375
1-310-471-9041 FAX

Publisher's Cataloging-in-Publication
Provided by Quality Books, Inc.
Gillespie, Larrian
    The gladiator diet : how to preserve peak health, sexual energy and a strong body at any age / Larrian Gillespie. – 1st ed.
    p. cm.
    Includes bibliographical references and index.
    LCCN: 00-110250
    ISBN: 0-9671317-4X

    1. Men--Health and hygiene. 2. Men--Nutrition.
    3. Physical fitness. I. Title

RA777.8.G55 2000   613.7'0449
                          QBI00-865

First Healthy Life Trade Printing: January 2001

Printed in the U.S.A.

10 9 8 7 6 5 4 3 2 1

The information found in this book is from the author's experiences and is not intended to replace medical advice. The author does not directly or indirectly dispense medical advice or prescribe the use of this nutritional program as a form of treatment. This publication is presented for informational purposes only. Before beginning this or any nutrition program you should consult with your physician.

Inside cover photo: Robert Cavalli, Still Moving Pictures
Book Design by: Barbara Hoorman
Cover Illustration ©Michael Sullivan, www.artboystudios.com

TABLE OF CONTENTS

DEDICATION

To Alexian

Always my daughter
now too my friend

ACKNOWLEDGMENTS

A book is never done without the help of so many. I would like to thank Jon Mathis and Tom Simon for burning the midnight oil to edit this book, and Barb Hoorman for her creative styling.

I have been blessed with so many friends, without whom I may not have made it through many a dark time. To Georganne and Ebar, Cher, Georgia, Emma, Carol and Rosemary, Carol and Mike, Carol and Ray, Carole and Tom, Sharon and Lois, Marilyn and Don, Myra and Alby, Dave and Susan, Lynda and Wayne, CJ, Roy and Gene, Pat, Perry, Elora, Lois, Mary and Jon, Deirdre and Gregg, Annie and Jack, Cate and in memorium—Cor, Helen, Richard, Helen, Gail and Grant, Jim and Anne, Judy and Mike, Bud and Sandy, Fay and Norvel, Meredyth and Shelly, Paula and Gerard, Füsun and Akif, thank you for showing me the meaning of unconditional love.

INTRODUCTION

The Hard Truth About Testosterone

It's a fact: men won't go to the doctor unless they fear something rather important is going to fall off. I should know. As one of the first women in the field of urology I specialized in treating men and women's "private parts," giving me a unique perspective as a physician into the healthcare concerns of men of all ages. While women routinely seek medical advice to improve their general health, men see a doctor, on average, 27 percent less often than women. Although men represent nearly half the population of the United States, they account for only 40 percent of physician's visits, according to the National Institutes of Health. No wonder men die about seven years sooner than women!

In all fairness, medicine has neglected the mid-life male, performing studies on healthy 22 year-olds to determine what is normal, then focusing on the "mature" man already affected by high cholesterol, lower testosterone levels, impotency and heart disease. But guys need to realize carrying around a waistline of 42 inches or greater at ANY age doubles their risk of impotency, heart disease, diabetes, high blood pressure, brittle bones and strokes.

An estimated 11 million Americans suffer type 2 Diabetes from being overweight, and more than half have high blood pressure, any of which can damage sensitive

> Although men represent nearly half the population of the United States, they account for only 40 percent of physician's visits

small blood vessels, including those that fill the penis. Men are developing brittle bones at an alarming rate, with one in every five victims of osteoporosis sporting a Y chromosome. But the real concern comes from increased cholesterol levels at a young age, which can result in the body producing inflammatory chemicals that rupture the linings of small blood vessels, leading to permanent tissue damage, including areas like the penis.

Exercise and the right diet help keep testosterone levels elevated

MALE MENOPAUSE

At the heart of all this are changes in testosterone levels. Unlike women, who expect a predictable timetable for ovarian failure, most men are unaware they will have a long but significant coast downhill to their own andropause, or male menopause. An estimated 30% of 65-year-old men have low testosterone levels by a young man's standards, yet medicine has not identified the "normal" levels for men at different ages. Exercise and the right diet help keep testosterone levels elevated...and that spells LOVE MACHINE at any age.

As in so many area of life, it's up to the woman to take subtle charge and make sure that her man remains healthy enough to see his children grow up and live long enough to be her lifelong champion and companion. In this book I will tell women how to banish a man's "Buddha Belly" caused by toxic stress and the wrong dietary advice. I will explain why a bloated waistline that raises estrogen levels in men can lead to impotency and heart disease, and I'll tell you how to keep him from "digging his grave with his teeth" every time he chows down on a low protein, high carbohydrate meal. And if you're worried about his virility,

I will reveal which foods and medical conditions will drop his testosterone and sperm counts lower than any number on a quarterback's jersey.

Ancient Roman gladiators epitomized the ultimate male...firm, fit and the object of adoring females. Although your guy doesn't need the "perfect physique" to be healthy, he can still avoid endangering his health and the welfare of your family by being overweight. The latest longevity stats used by the insurance industry predict that anyone who had reached age 50 at the millennium has a one in two chance of living to 100. But that doesn't hold for more than 65% of American men age 25 and above who are overweight. Obesity has reached epidemic proportions in the United States, but your man doesn't have to become part of this statistic if you feed him The Gladiator Diet.[1]

To date, more than 30 million men have unnecessarily taken Viagra for erectile dysfunction (ED) caused by reversible conditions.

It's time to become fearless and help him own the power of natural health.

CHAPTER 1
Firm, Fit and Fearless

If doctors were after-hours lingerie models, men wouldn't need to be dragged in by their ears for treatment of any medical problem where there wasn't serious jeopardy of something important "falling off." The same guy who wouldn't dream of letting his car go 3,000 miles without an oil change probably can't tell you when he last had his blood pressure checked or his cholesterol level monitored. Yet the average man has a 1-in-4 chance of having high blood pressure and heart disease before the age of 60, and a 1-in-12 chance of developing diabetes, which triples his risk of impotency, especially after age 50.[2] But in an even more startling report, doctors have found that men with a waistline of 42 inches instead of a trim, firm 32 inch waist, are twice as likely to develop erectile dysfunction, (ED), regardless of age.[3] Seems like that size label on his Levi's may be telling women more than he wants them to know!

Packing on the pounds, especially around his waistline, can expose more than a butt crack on a man. Fat cells in this region are especially handy at converting testosterone into estradiol, the active form of estrogen.[4,5] This female hormone, in turn, becomes a bit "butch" and starts knocking testosterone out of various cellular receptor sites, sending signals to the brain to lower testosterone production. In no time, his cholesterol and blood sugar start to rise, his hairstyle takes on the tonsured look of a monk and he's chemically neutered by a hormonal sucker punch.[6] And if losing that loving feeling isn't enough to get the attention of either one of you, he could be seeing stars by getting KO'd with an increased risk of heart attacks.[7]

It's a sobering thought...but impotency may be one of the earliest signs of asymptomatic heart disease. Atherosclerosis, or hardening of the arteries (including the delicate ones in the penis) can begin as early as age 30, when testosterone levels begin to change, especially if a man is overweight. By the time he reaches 40, a man runs a greater than 12% risk of experiencing impotency, increasing to nearly 47% by the age of 65.[8] Insulin is the culprit behind all this damage to the family jewels. It's the hormone responsible for handling the sugar produced from carbohydrates...you know, the stuff he loads up on before running a marathon or biking in the Tour de France.

Impotency may be one of the earliest signs of asymptomatic heart disease

CARBOHYDRATE SENSITIVITY SYNDROME

Carbohydrates are divided into two categories: complex and simple. (Table 1) Think of these foods as starches and sugars which vary in particle size. A simple carbohydrate has very small, fine particles, (as in sugar or refined, processed foods) while complex carbs are natural, large molecules,(as in lentils, squash and broccoli). Most large molecules are absorbed more slowly because all food has to be broken down into the smallest particle. That's why small, simple carbohydrates shoot right into your blood stream. However, some complex carbohydrates, like corn, contain more natural sugars and can enter the blood just as quickly, acting like a simple carbohydrate in triggering your body's insulin response.

Glucose is the fuel which enables the mitochondria to act like little thermonuclear reactors, splitting off electrons which generate energy for cellular function. Every organ in your body requires

SIMPLE CARBOHYDRATES		TABLE 1
JAMS	JELLIES	SUGAR/FRUCTOSE
HONEY	CORN /TABLE SYRUP	MOLASSES
PIES	CANDY	CAKES
COOKIES	PASTRIES	SODA POP

COMPLEX CARBOHYDRATES
— HIGH FIBER FOODS —

BREADS	PASTA	CEREALS
FLOURS	BARLEY	RICE
PEAS	BEANS	LENTILS
POTATOES	CORN	FRUITS
NUTS	SEEDS	

glucose just to function. Glucose is either burned immediately or stored in the form of glycogen in the liver and muscles as emergency reserves. Once these sites are full, the rest is stored as fat.

Insulin keeps blood glucose levels from rising too high by pushing glucose, amino acids and free fatty acids out of the bloodstream and into cells as quickly as possible for immediate use. Another hormone, glucagon, prevents insulin from being too efficient and causing hypoglycemia. Both hormones are secreted by the pancreas. When he eats carbohydrates, the petite particles are absorbed from the small intestine into the bloodstream, elevating his glucose levels. Like the newest vacuum cleaner, insulin "beats, it sweeps, it cleans" his blood of glucose by shoving it into cells. Any excess is stored in fat cells. As if to add insult to injury, insulin signals previously stored fat to stay put. Now excess free fatty acids are sent to the liver where they are converted into cholesterol. Remember, hormones are the chemical internet within his body that directs the breakdown and buildup of new cells. When testosterone levels are low or out of balance, insulin levels rise and more cells break down, giving men that haggard look of accelerated aging.

Glucagon, on the other hand, is stimulated by proteins and a low glucose level. It has the laudable job of promoting the breakdown of stored fat in order to achieve equilibrium. This is a GOOD thing! It's also capable of helping the liver convert amino acids derived from protein into glucose in case of starvation. The best news is that once glucagon levels are elevated, they remain so for at least four hours.[9]

Alteration in a man's sensitivity to insulin cripples its effectiveness in lowering his blood sugar, forcing his pancreas to work overtime making more and more insulin just to do the same job. You already know that insulin aids in storing fat. This makes it MORE efficient at storing excess glucose as fat as it becomes LESS efficient at lowering his blood glucose levels. Bah-dah bing he's developed a carbohydrate sensitivity which adds fat while knocking testosterone levels down a peg. This means that a couple of the mobsters on the Sopranos are probably a quart low in testosterone, but I'll let someone else tell them that! Metabolic Syndrome X is characterized by men who have two or more of the following conditions: insulin resistance with resulting high insulin levels, elevated lipids (especially triglycerides), abdominal obesity, coronary artery disease and hypertension. Not surprisingly, it has been found to be associated with borderline testosterone deficiency.[10, 11]

Low testosterone affects serotonin

HE'S NOT IN THE MOOD

Lower testosterone levels not only prevent sperm

from winning an Olympic swim match but affect another hormone, serotonin, which is important in controlling his mood. The male who eats a low protein, low fat diet, deprives his brain of the ability to make serotonin, which results in depression and even headaches. Low serotonin levels signal the thyroid to slow down his metabolism, which can cause tiredness, hair loss, weight gain and low sex drive. Stress and high carbohydrate diets add to this pyramid of hormonal imbalances.

When testosterone levels drop, so does the release of cholecystokinin, a hormone produced by the pancreas which signals his gallbladder to empty. Cholecystokinin makes a man feel full or satiated, especially when he has saturated fat in his diet. But when the ratio of testosterone to estrogen gets out of balance, your desperado experiences a substantial delay in gallbladder emptying and just doesn't feel full as soon as he should. As a result, portion size increases, and he craves more calories. Changes in his ability to handle carbohydrates adds another wallop. As blood sugar rises, so does his hunger quotient and any cholecystokinin released not only fails to signal he's full, but paradoxically increases his appetite.[12] Now he's eating like Jabba the Hut – and with all that fat, he's converting testosterone into estrogen. Overnight he mysteriously understands how women wrap that towel around their heads when leaving the shower.

Fat cells convert testosterone into estrogen

NO, HE WON'T MENSTRUATE

Surprised that a guy's body makes estrogen? Most people are unaware that males normally produce between 2-60 pg/ml of estradiol, the active form of estrogen, or that fat contains an enzyme, called aromatase, which fat cells use to convert testosterone into estradiol. So the more fat cells a man carries, the more little hormone factories are manufacturing estradiol in his body. Not only does this increase his clotting ability and risk for a heart attack or stroke, but it has also been known to trigger an irresistible urge to go shoe shopping. Elevated estradiol levels stimulate his liver to juice up its hydroelectric plant, (in the form of CP450 enzymes), to clear excess estradiol from his body and improve his testosterone

A TRIP THROUGH YOUR DIGESTIVE TRACT

Think of your stomach as a washing machine. You "load" it with food, which has not yet been carefully sorted; that is, proteins, carbohydrates and fat all get tossed in together. Your stomach next adds the "pre-treatment enzymes" and detergent, called hormones. Gastrin stimulates the release of serotonin, histamine, hydrochloric acid and acetylcholine, which cause the stomach to contract. The enzyme pepsin efficiently seeks out any of the aromatic amino acids in your food, (tryptophan, tyrosine and phenylalanine), and chops them off from the rest of the proteins. The "cycle" changes and the emulsified food is spun into the duodenum, or first part of the small intestine.

Now the pancreas takes charge. It secretes chymotrypsin to remove any residual bits of these amino acids, and also release cholecystokinin to contract your gall bladder. This makes you feel full. The contracting gallbladder releases bile, which helps break up carbohydrates and fats. The pancreas then dumps insulin into the bloodstream to handle sugars extracted from carbohydrates. Amino acids found in proteins are then used to make neurotransmitters. When blood sugar starts to fall too low, the pancreas releases glucagon to prevent hypoglycemia. During all this time, the liver is directing your metabolism based upon the efficiency rating of your digestion. Finally, the pancreas ejects bicarbonate and "rinses" the food, stopping all the action of the stomach's enzymes. It performs this last cycle before sending it to the "dryer", the rest of your small bowel, where any excess water and tiny nutrients left over are absorbed into the bloodstream as the final cleanup from digestion. The entire cycle normally takes about two hours. (Figure 1)

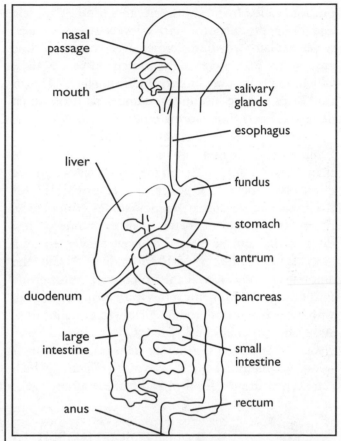

FIGURE I
the digestive
system

to estradiol ratio. But several things, like alcohol, marijuana and depleted zinc levels can make those enzymes behave like water in a race car's fuel line. This can shift the balance in favor of estrogen, which sabotages his ability to maintain an adequate testosterone level.

IN A BIND

Not all of his testosterone is free to circulate. In fact, most of it is bound to Sex Hormone Binding Globulin (SHBG) proteins in his blood. Estrogen increases the amount of this protein, which in turn gobbles up his testosterone, leaving only a small portion, called free testosterone, to stimulate muscle and bone production. SHBG levels rise with age, which explains why testosterone levels start to decline around age 30. Interestingly, protein lowers SHBG, which results in more bioactive testosterone.[13] This in turn helps to keep insulin levels under control, which deters his body from storing fat.

Even in the "Baywatch Bodies" state of California, where there are more juice bars and gyms than burger joints, 60% of men are overweight or clinically obese.[14] Obesity is responsible for hypertension, gallstones, kidney stones, impotency, heart attacks and diabetes,—just to name a few diseases that can be allayed or even prevented by a guy losing as little as 5-10 pounds.[15-18,19] Cut the amount of body fat available to convert testosterone into estrogen, and men capture pure hormonal gold, with more free testosterone available to enhance their strength, potency and energy...just like a true gladiator! So if you're ready to help polish his inner hood ornament, let me show you the factors which can keep your man fit, firm and fearless at any age.

GLADIATOR GUIDELINES

The average man has a 1-in- 4 chance of suffering high blood pressure and heart disease before the age of 60, and a 1-in-12 chance of developing diabetes, which triples his risk of impotency, especially after age 50.   FACT

A waistline of 42 inches carries with it twice the risk of developing impotency or erectile dysfunction (ED) regardless of his age.   FACT

Fat converts testosterone into estrogen, which increases a man's risk for a heart attack, stroke and impotency.   FACT

Losing as little as 10 pounds can dramatically increase a man's testosterone levels.   FACT

CHAPTER 2
Buddha Belly Syndrome:
A Road Sign for Impotency,
Diabetes and Heart Disease

A healthy weight is not determined by numbers on a scale, but by where fats are stored in the body. More importantly, not all fat cells behave alike. The most metabolically active fats lurk like some vile creature in the deep dark of the abdomen. As a result, a man can look very fit but be fairly fat. Genetics plays a role in this, but scientists are acknowledging that a man's hormone balance dictates where he puts on fat.

FAT'S GOTTEN UNDER YOUR SKIN

Both visceral and subcutaneous fat have the same composition—75% fatty acids and 25% glycerol, a type of alcohol. While the fat cells inside his abdomen are smaller than their distant cousins on his hips, these little creatures are more active, releasing fatty acids into the blood stream while picking up additional fat for storage. Because they snuggle up to the blood vessels surrounding all his internal organs, they can deliver fatty acids to tissue with little constraint. As a result, the liver is bathed with blood that is very high in free fatty acids, which leads to the production of less of the good cholesterol, called high density lipoproteins (HDL) and more of the bad or low density cholesterol (LDL). Any tissue surrounded by fatty acids is less able to remove insulin from the bloodstream, and more fat gets stored. The more intra-abdominal fat, the higher the insulin levels.[20]

FIGURE 2

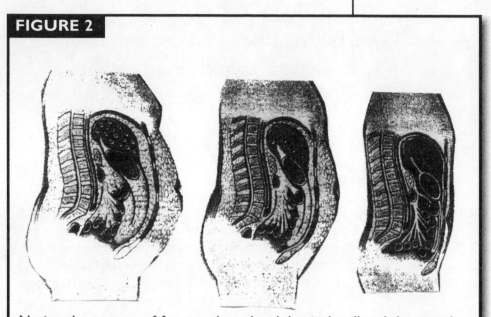

Notice the amount of fat stored on the abdominal wall and deep inside the belly.

THE OMENTRUM

As a surgeon, I constantly encountered the omentum, a fatty apron of tissue between the lining of the abdomen and the bowel that keeps them from sticking together. This organ also acts as a giant sponge within a guy's abdomen, soaking up any fluid that comes in contact with it...blood, electrolyte solutions, or lymph. It has the additional ability to concentrate neurochemicals, (especially norepinephrine, epinephrine and dopamine from your intestines) in its venous blood and tissue.[21] This makes it a very active biological organ, capable of mobilizing fat in response to insulin and cortisol. This organ is able to swell and enlarge when faced with excess amounts of these neurotransmitters, which are found in red meat and manufactured from

The omentrum mobilizes fat

foods high in the amino acids tryptophan, tyrosine and tyramine. If you've fed him a meal and watched him tug at his belt before he's left the table, it's his omentum working overtime.

THE RULES OF FAT DISTRIBUTION

Just how the body stores fat is a bit complex, but it's also crucial to understanding metabolism. By measuring the turnover of fat tissue triglycerides, researchers found the body first tries to store fats in the omentum and retroperitoneal areas (the deep parts of his pelvis), then in the subcutaneous regions of the abdomen and finally in the subcutaneous femoral area on the thigh.[4] As fat grows in the abdomen, hormones panic. Cortisol climbs and testosterone drops, a result of signals sent along the information highway connecting the hypothalamus, pituitary and adrenals. Adrenaline is a protein-burning hormone which can waste away his lean muscle mass and increase his insulin resistance. The more muscle cells he depletes, the less storage sites are left for sugar. Fat cells, under the direction of cortisol and insulin, promote fat storage by expressing lipoprotein lipase, a fat accumulating enzyme. Abdominal fat cells pack more in per square inch, and have a greater blood supply, along with more nerve connections, to detour fats to their area. In short, aging, depression, stress, chronic dieting, smoking and excess alcohol intake shift the balance from the fat mobilizing couple (testosterone and growth hormone) to the fat accumulating couple (cortisol and insulin).

LOCATION LOCATION LOCATION

Like real estate, everything about fat boils down to location. Fat cells, called adipocytes, can store more or less fat dependent upon their position in the body. Intra-abdominal or visceral cells are the sumo wrestlers of fat storage, enlarging to gargantuan size when we put our bodies under chronic stress. These lard buckets have more receptors for glucocorticoids than peripheral fat cells, allowing them to preferentially direct the fat traffic to their sites.[22] Insulin causes fluid retention by making a man more sensitive to salt and expands the tissue surrounding these cells. Cortisol speeds up the intestine's ability to transport fat through your bloodstream to fat storage sites. This makes it harder for fat depots to clear out the products of fat breakdown—glycerol and free fatty acids. This prevents further mobilization of fat.[23] You can almost hear those fat cells squishing when he chomps down on a "stress relieving" bag of potato chips.

Abdominal fat is why men develop insulin resistance and a lower testosterone level

THE SENSITIVE SIDE OF FAT

Abdominal fat has a significantly stronger relationship with insulin sensitivity than peripheral non-abdominal fat, making men with an android or Buddha Belly shape more insulin resistant than those with fat on their legs. Scientists say abdominal fat may be a major reason why men develop insulin resistance and a lower testosterone level.[24]

With excess fat hiding in his abdomen, there is an increased risk for prostate, pancreatic and gallbladder cancer. This is due to elevated levels of circulating estrogens created from alterations of male sex steroids in fat tissue, combined with decreased levels of sex hormone-binding globulin (SHBG).[25,26] As insulin levels go up, the testicles decrease the production of male sex hormones—testosterone and androstene-dione—and infertility and impotency occurs. Meals high in carbohydrates stimulate higher levels of insulin which in turn causes a rise in estrogens. Obese men with infertility and impotency are probably helping their disease along with every meal they eat. The great news is all this can be reversed by simple weight loss. [27]

The bad news is even a normal weight can be unhealthy in some men. Scientists measured the hidden fat within the abdomens of men of normal weight, using computerized tomography, or a CAT scan. Instead of weight, researchers studied the amount of body fat. Using a body mass index (BMI, which is your weight divided by your height squared) of 25 as normal, they were able to determine that men should have a desirable waist measurement around 33 inches regardless of their height, if they don't want to raise their risk factors for impotency, heart disease and diabetes.[28] Even with a BMI of only 27, or about 10 pounds of extra fat, men were found to significantly lower their testosterone levels.[13] The swing of the needle on a scale means very little if a man stuffs most of his fat into his abdomen.[29]

Buddha bellies are the result of age, pure and simple. Growth hormone, which directs fat metabolism and helps build muscles, takes an elevator ride to the basement and men start to lose fat-burning muscle mass. Once this happens, your gladiator's ability to burn calories falls, and any excess food that finds its way down his digestive tracts gets sidelined into fat. As he replaces lean muscle with fat, he keeps lowering his energy efficiency rating. Total body weight goes up and now the problems really start.

10 pounds of extra fat lowers testosterone

THE CHINESE CONNECTION

This information crosses all cultural lines. Studies on healthy Chinese men and women with heavy torsos showed they were at a higher risk of cardiovascular disease even though they weren't technically fat.[30] Deep intra-abdominal fat correlated with higher blood pressure, glucose, triglyceride and low HDL levels – all known to put men at increased risk for heart disease. So even eating a traditional oriental diet can't change the impact central body fat has on survival.

INSULIN: THE EVIL TWIN

When guys gain fat a not-so-funny thing happens to their insulin levels – they go up – and that results in more fat storage. Small amounts of insulin lower blood sugar, but if insulin sticks around, it turns men into porkers. Cholesterol levels jump and the good triglycerides tank. High, sustained insulin levels accelerate the formation of blood clots, and that makes your buckaroo more susceptible to strokes and heart attacks. As a final kick in the pants, too much insulin eventually stiffens his blood vessels, causing hypertension and impotency.

RUBBING OUT THE BUDDHA BELLY

So how do you convince your man he is growing a Buddha Belly? The most reliable indicator seems to be his waist-to-hip ratio (WHR), which indicates where most of his fat is located. The next important road sign is the circumference of his waist. To find his WHR, measure around the fullest part of his buttocks (this is his hip measurement) and then measure his waist (the narrowest part of his torso between his lowest rib and his iliac crest or hip bone.) Simply divide his waist by his hip measurement. A healthy ratio is less than 1 with an ideal ratio around 0.9. A WHR greater than 1.04 is characteristic of upper body obesity. Men with this body shape have more bloated fat cells which lead to higher sustained insulin levels. This make insulin less effective at lowering his blood sugar and more efficient at producing large amounts of female sex hormones. In addition, men with this body shape have elevated plasma lipid profiles and are at a high risk of developing non-insulin dependent diabetes and coronary heart disease.[28, 31-33]

So what is directing all these changes? A wedge-shaped gland called the hypothalamus.

THIS IS HIS BRAIN ON PATROL

Located at the base of the third ventricle in the brain, the hypothalamus acts as the "Great and Wonderful Wizard" of his hormones, sending signals to the pituitary, which in turn barks orders to the other endocrine glands – the adrenals, thyroid and testicles.

When the hypothalamus detects that testosterone levels are too low, it sends an e-mail to his pituitary to release a hormone called gondaotrophin-releasing hormone, or GnRH. Like a chain letter, several other hormones, called leutenizing hormone (LH) and follicle-stimulating hormone (FSH) get passed along to his bloodstream in hourly intervals. These hormones stimulate cells in the testicles to produce testosterone, which in turn will let the hypothalamus know when levels are back to normal.

However, sometimes the cells in his testicles get a bit cranky...okay, they have a temper tantrum, and don't want to cooperate. His testosterone levels drop, even though his testicles are perfectly normal. This alerts his adrenals, which swing into action releasing cortisol, the stress hormone, which in turn tells fat cells to open up their expandable tanks and take on more storage. Fat metabolism jumps and those fat cells which have a greater blood supply turn into gluttons. Unfortunately, these are the very ones that surround the bowel and line his abdominal cavity giving him the Buddha Belly shape.

FIGURE 3

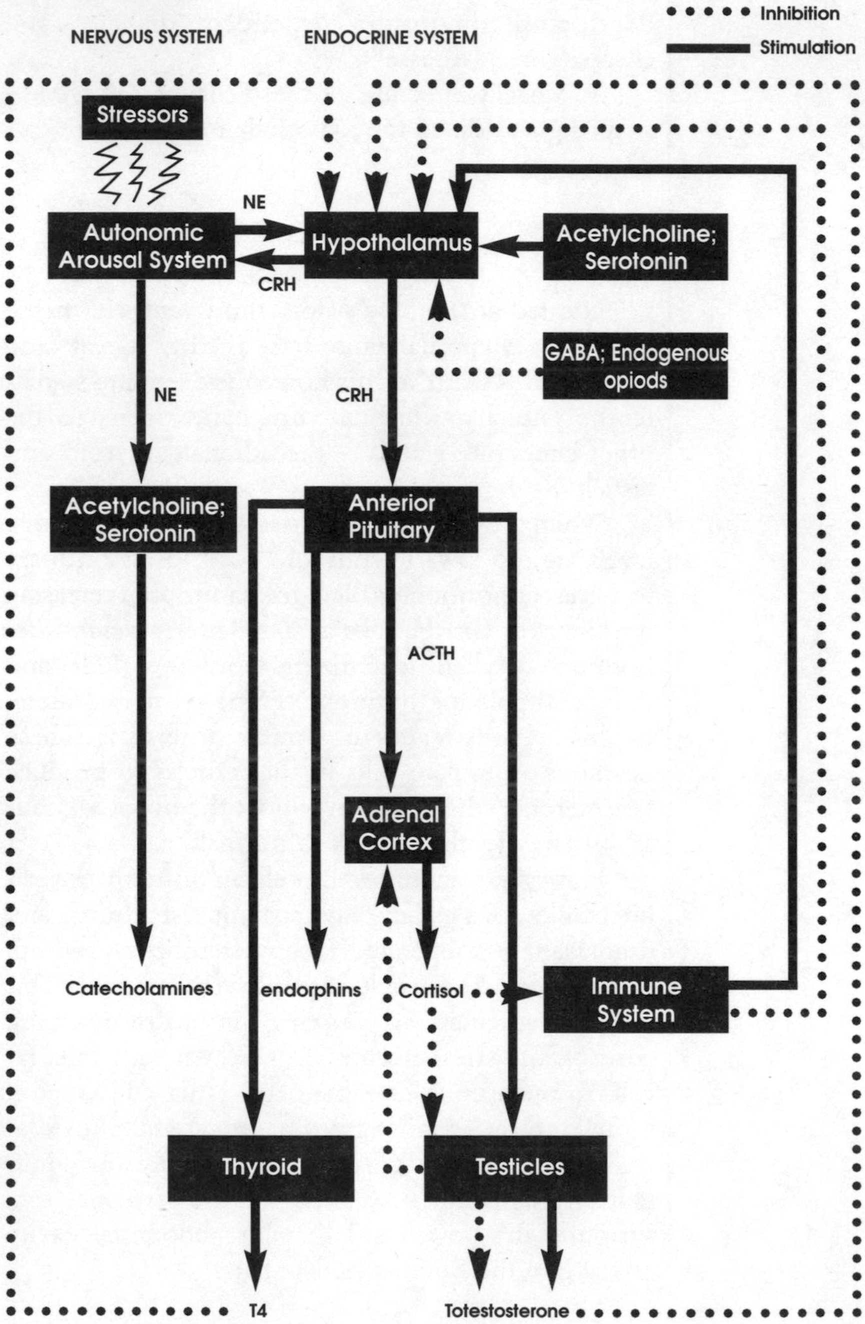

NERVOUS SYSTEM   ENDOCRINE SYSTEM

• • • • • Inhibition
━━━━━ Stimulation

Stressors

NERVOUS SYSTEM

Autonomic Arousal System

NE

Hypothalamus

CRH

Acetylcholine; Serotonin

GABA; Endogenous opiods

NE

CRH

Acetylcholine; Serotonin

Anterior Pituitary

ACTH

Adrenal Cortex

Catecholamines   endorphins   Cortisol   Immune System

Thyroid   Testicles

T4   Totestosterone

THE THREAT TO HIS HEALTH

Diabetes strikes more than eight million people a year, while an additional eight million remain undiagnosed with non-insulin dependent diabetes (NIDDM or type II).[34] Astonishingly, an estimated 20 million persons meet the criteria for impaired glucose tolerance, a condition in which blood glucose levels are higher than normal but not high enough to be diagnosed as diabetes. Hyperglycemia and impaired glucose tolerance, as seen when a man's hormones get out of balance, convey a significant risk for heart disease and full-blown diabetes.[35] Not surprisingly, it's the sugar extracted by his stomach from the foods he eats that result in the high glucose levels seen after eating in early undiagnosed diabetes. In fact, the first sign of diabetes is elevated glucose for several hours after a meal.[36]

It seems cholesterol numbers can be deceiving. Excess sugar can result in cholesterol being deposited as a liquid plaque within the blood vessels feeding the heart, especially in men. This type of plaque doesn't block the vessels like a column, and can't be detected by treadmills or angiograms. Not surprisingly, the formation of these liquid-filled cavities is aggravated by elevated insulin levels. Once they burst, they fill the entire blood vessel with a core of cholesterol, making them a silent killer in men with hormonal imbalances. You've probably already guessed the two most significant risk factors for developing either diabetes or heart disease—smoking and abdominal obesity.

AND NOW FOR THE BUDDHA BELLY AWARDS

So what are the risk factors for gaining abdominal or central fat? Men who eat large amounts of saturated fat, especially from meat, frequently drink alcohol, smoke, or have gained a lot of weight since the age of 18 have twice as much chance of winning the "Buddha Belly Award" than men who eat a diet high in vegetables and exercise.[37] Gaining weight does more than make him look fat—it can endanger his health, shorten his life span and even trigger life-threatening diseases. Now for the good news. If you look at all the illnesses listed in Table 2, each and every one can be modified by losing that unhappy Buddha Belly. If you're ready to change your man's lifestyle and want him to be healthy and fit for the rest of your lives, let me show you how simple it is to help him lose the weight and keep it off. He won't need pills or surgery and you can both end up saving a lot of money. Interested? Then let's get started!

TABLE 2 — BUDDHA BELLY DAMAGE FACTORS

- Arthritis
- Hypertension
- Cancer of the prostate, gallbladder, kidneys
- Incontinence
- Coronary Heart Disease
- Kidney failure
- Chronic lung disease
- Kidney stones
- Diabetes

- Gallstones
- Sleep apnea
- Stroke
- Irritable Bowel Syndrome
- Migraines
- Depression
- Infertility
- Osteoporosis
- Bloating
- Cataracts

CHAPTER 3
The
Gladiator Diet

If chariots fit in drive-throughs, a gladiator's order might go something like this: double cheese roast oxen burger on barley bread, extra onions sauteed in olive oil, topped with beans and vegetables. Throw in wine, nuts and figs and you have a traditional athletic meal served in ancient Rome to men who were expending about 3000 calories a day through exercise.[38] Hardly today's scenario, where fast foods and television viewing have been implicated in the current epidemic of obesity in the United States.[39]

In recent years, scientists have recognized that fat tissue on a man's body is a source of estrogen, allowing androstenedione, an adrenal hormone, to be converted to estrone, a very active form of estrogen. This flags the hypothalamus to slow production of testosterone, which in turn, causes a more sustained rise in insulin. Blood sugar levels go up and fat cells start packing away sugar like it was their last meal. And if he's eating 750 to 1000 calories at a time, a guy's blood insulin and glucose levels can stay high for up to five hours. This can set the stage for heart disease, hypertension, impotence, obesity, cataracts and the signs of aging.

This delayed but prolonged rise in insulin and glucose inhibits the release of glucagon, the hormone that helps a man to burn previously stored fat. Within thirty minutes of eating protein, glucagon levels start to rise, peaking at two hours.[40] In fact, glucagon can stay elevated in blood for several hours after a protein rich meal. This gives his body plenty of time to use the fat around his waist and hips as the energy source to fuel his brain.

ALL CARBOHYDRATES ARE NOT CREATED EQUAL

Since 1927, scientists have known that different carbohydrates with the same nutrient composition produce different glucose responses in the body.[41] A "sugar profile" was developed for each food enabling doctors to predict the effect of digestion on the availability of glucose in the body. By comparing other foods to the glucose response achieved by eating just a few slices of white bread, a glycemic index of carbohydrate metabolism was established.[42-44] This gave doctors the freedom to exchange carbohydrate choices for diabetic patients without risking big swings in their blood glucose levels.

Not all foods, however, are created equal. The particle size of a particular food and the degree of gelatinization or gumminess which it undergoes when cooked affects how much glucose or sugar can be obtained by digestion. Rice is a good example of a food that can vary markedly depending upon the amylose or starch content. The higher the amylose, the greater the gelatinization and the lower the glycemic index (GI).[45] The more processed a food becomes, the smaller the particle size and the greater the GI. That's why bread, french fries, corn chips, canned pea soup, angel food cake and Cheerios™, all highly processed foods, have almost identical GI values and insulin responses.[46]

PROTEIN POWER

Much has been made about the ability of protein to decrease blood sugar levels when added to a carbohydrate meal. The exact effect, however, depends upon both the type and amount of protein and the medical condition of the person eating the combination. In men with normal testosterone levels and non-insulin dependent diabetics (NIDDM), protein stimulates insulin secretion but not glucose, which causes a drop in blood sugar. However, it requires a LOT of protein to do this. Let me give you an example: Four slices of white bread contain 50 gm of carbohydrate which acts like 3 tablespoons of corn syrup in his body. It would take 50 gm of protein (that's 12 ounces or 3 chicken breasts) to cancel out that bread.[47] If a man were an insulin-dependent diabetic, he would increase rather than decrease his blood sugar levels by adding that much protein to his meal.

Protein, however, does stimulate the production of glucagon which, along with cholecystokinin, can help to decrease a man's meal size by signaling that he's full.[48] When protein is eaten first, it stimulates glucagon, cholecystokinin and the hormone motilin, which jump starts the gastric wave to empty the stomach.

FAT FACTS

The addition of fat to a carbohydrate creates a greater insulin response

Fat, especially saturated fat, slows digestion in the stomach. It also impedes the activity of the small bowel in propelling food along the digestive tract.[49] Delayed gastric emptying lowers his blood sugar response to a meal. A lot has been made about eating specific ratios of fat and protein to maintain normal glucose levels. This Zone approach flies in the face of current research. If you put 25 gms of fat or 2 1/2 tablespoons of butter on white bread it will have no effect on preventing the sugar rise in normal people.[50] The addition of fat to a carbohydrate gives you the same blood sugar response as if you ate the carbohydrate alone. And worse, there's a greater insulin response. This is not good, as the longer insulin stays around, the more his tissue resists releasing fat. So combining ratios of fat and protein with carbohydrates can reduce his blood sugar response but only if relatively large amounts of either are used.[51]

Snacking on "macho meals" keeps his insulin levels down

MIX IT UP

When a man eats a "mixed meal" of protein, carbohydrate and fat, the blood sugar rise can be predicted from the glycemic index of the carbohydrate alone. This is significant, because only by choosing foods that are low in their ability to turn his body into a sugar cube can you help him achieve a more normal insulin response.[52] Furthermore, by eating a breakfast full of low glycemic carbs, he can lower his insulin response to a standard lunch meal by as much as 30%.[53] An added benefit of eating low GI foods is a normal bowel movement, as nearly 20% of the undigested starch from these foods will be metabolized in the colon, acting as additional fiber in his diet.

GRAZE OR GORGE

Another way to keep his blood sugar under control is to get him to eat several small meals instead of one or two big meals. I call these "macho meals," because of their results. Snacking on small 350 calorie "macho meals" can keep his insulin levels down, which in turn lowers his cholesterol.[54] As an added bonus, small meals relieve the stress on his body, as evidenced by lower cortisol and cholesterol levels.[55, 56] By simply reducing the rate at which he presents food to his digestive tract he can dramatically reduce the rate of lipids or fats appearing in his blood, regardless of what he eats.[57, 58]

Eating all his calories at one meal overloads the

circuitry of his body's digestive process and causes a metabolic "blackout," which has devastating effects on his circulation, not to mention his waistline. But if he snacks on five to six meals a day with the same amount of calories, he can maintain an even level of sugar and fats in his blood. By spreading the calories of a meal throughout the course of a day his body will trigger a counter regulatory mechanism that sends growth hormone levels up for four hours after each meal. Remember, the more growth hormone around, the more he burns fat instead of muscle, which can boost his testosterone level.

Men and women's bodies can tolerate a rise in fat levels between 10 to 30% and still keep the insulin, glucose and corticosterone levels low, but if our food contains more than 30% fat we end up with elevated blood sugar levels and store more fat.[59] By eating multiple meals and spreading the calories, our bodies can handle the occasional fat load in excess of 30%.[55]

CAN ONE MEAL AFFECT THE NEXT?

Men's bodies can be downright stingy when it comes to letting insulin out of their wallet if they eat meals closer together. The Staub-Traugott effect explains why the closeness of one meal to the next determines the blood sugar response to the second meal. The closer together the meals are, the better the glucose tolerance and the less insulin the body needs to keep blood sugar in check.

Fiber lowers blood glucose levels

The amount of fiber in a meal can also affect the burst of insulin he releases when faced with the next meal. Fiber, by its sheer ability to slow down digestion, can lower blood glucose levels. High fiber soups can significantly suppress hunger and reduce the amount of calories desired in the next meal, especially if he eats a "chunky hearty man" soup.[60] But this is not the main reason the composition of one meal affects the next one's ability to elevate his blood sugar. In a study of mixed meals with different fiber contents but the same glycemic carbohydrate content, researchers found that a dinner composed of low glycemic carbohydrates improved anyone's carbohydrate tolerance for breakfast.[61] It's like having overdraft protection built into his carbohydrate checkbook.

Folate lowers homocysteine levels

THE FRENCH PARADOX

Now that you have explained to him the advantages of "macho meals" you've understood a paradigm that stumped researchers for years, called The French Paradox. It seems our French relations, who helped us win independence from England, may also be helping us lose our fat. Although the French eat more saturated fat and smoke and drink alcohol, they have 40% fewer heart attacks than Americans.

So how do they do it?
• The French consume moderate amounts of alcohol, especially red wine, usually with meats
• The French eat more fresh fruit and vegetables
• The French eat less red meat
• The French consume more cheese and less whole milk
• The French use more olive oil and less butter or lard, and they take longer to eat meals and snack less on high carbohydrate foods

Eating a diet high in fruit and vegetables offers his body high levels of folate, which lowers plasma homocysteine levels, a dietary byproduct of animal protein. Even mild to moderate elevation in blood values of this amino acid is a strong risk factor for atherosclerosis, clogging up arteries to the penis, brain, heart and limbs.[62] In a study of the French diet, researchers found that few French adults met American USDA recommendations. Only 14% of those studied got their fat levels below 30% and less than 4% of the French ate less than 10% of <u>that</u> fat as saturated fat. In contrast, 90% of them had a more diverse diet. Much like the advice given by any financial advisor, diversity in your man's food choices seems to be an important factor in protecting his life's assets against fluctuations in the energy consumption market.

Although the French are not known for their exercise clubs, their lifestyles are naturally more active. They live in small villages, they walk a lot, and their lives don't revolve around cars and malls. They shop every day and carry home fresh food and rarely fix meals from cans. Foods are available seasonally, instead of put into cold storage for later use, which affects the nutritional content of the food. Cars are a luxury, so the French end up walking with weighted packages several times a day. Meals in restaurants are expensive, so more socialization is done at wine bars or bistros where a single dish may be consumed over an hour of friendly conversation. The French are more aware than Americans of the importance of choosing foods that protect against heart disease and cancer, such as fruits and vegetables, especially tomatoes, which can protect against tumors of the digestive and respiratory tracts.[63,64] But most of all, the French understand the importance of breakfast.[65] When you sleep, your body is essentially fasting. But your brain is working overtime using up stores of glycogen to keep your neuroelectric grid lit. That's why the first meal of the day is called "break(ing the) fast." By not eating breakfast, you force your body to break down muscle to provide glycogen for your brain. This signals a famine, which alerts your body to store whatever food you eat as fat.

The French understand the importance of breakfast

FUDGING WITH FAT

Numerous studies show a positive link between

dietary fat and fatness. However, only recently have researchers focused on the type of fat as well as the amount in our diets. It seems the amount of fat intake can only explain about 2% of the fat snuggled under his skin and hiding inside his frame.[66] Lowering saturated fat intake can have a dramatic effect on lowering cholesterol, especially LDL, or the bad low-density cholesterol.[67] It seems fudging your fat intake by substituting more mono-unsaturated fats like olive oil can result not only in weight loss but a much better cholesterol and insulin response.[68] Even a handful of peanuts, which are rich in oleic acid, can make a difference in a man's risk for heart disease.[69]

Butter has gotten a bad rap. While palm, coconut and olive oil caused the highest concentration of cholesterol in the blood, butter produced an intermediate response in the blood, liver and gallbladder and ·was not linked to gallstone formation.[70] Butter also contains buteric acid, which helps your stud muffin absorb nutrients from his food. So even if you're watching his cholesterol, don't nag him if he eats a little unsalted butter.

Butter helps him absorb nutrients

DIGGING HIS GRAVE WITH HIS OWN TEETH

Unfortunately, all these facts fly in the face of the very diet his doctor or other experts may be suggesting. The current recommended diet for men emphasizes substituting carbohydrates for saturated fat without concern for their ability to raise his blood sugar level.[71] Low fat, high carbohydrate diets increase insulin concentration in his blood, which can raise his risk for heart disease and impotency. The more insulin resistant he becomes, the greater the negative effects on insulin, glucose and cholesterol if he cheats and eats a high-carbohydrate, low fat diet. Studies bear this out.

Two diets were tested using the following

composition of carbohydrates, fat and protein: Group 1 ate a 60/25/15 ratio and Group 2 consumed a 40/45/15 diet. That's right—45% fat. The ratios of mono, poly and saturated fat were the same. As predicted, those who replaced fat with carbs had a marked decrease in the good high-density cholesterol with an overall elevation in LDL /HDL ratios to above 4.0, which is considered dangerous.[72,73] This is not an isolated study, but rather consistent with numerous large epidemiological studies of men and their risk for heart disease.[74,15] The answer seems clear: low fat, high carbohydrate diets can cause dangerous changes in his health, especially if he is insulin resistant. He's digging his own grave with his teeth every time he loads up on high glycemic carbs. It just makes sense to cut saturated fat in his diet by increasing mono-unsaturated fats and low glycemic carbs instead of reaching for those potato chips. And if you want him to maintain his weight loss, mono-unsaturated fatty acids are key.[75] Afraid he'll start whimpering about letting go of saturated fats? Here's a tip: decrease the quantity at each meal and he won't even notice.

FAT AND CANCER

Everyone blames fats for causing cancer. Just look at the diseases listed in Table 3.

While saturated fat can increase your risk for cancer, there is little evidence that mono-unsaturated fats affect these tumors. As Americans cut down on butter and dairy, they substituted n-6-polyunsaturated oils-vegetable oils, which are thought to promote cancer.

As a result, prostate and colon cancer have become more common.[76] The higher concentration of fats and phospholipids as well as increased levels of estrogen produced from the conversion of body fat to estradiol is to blame. No greater proof of the

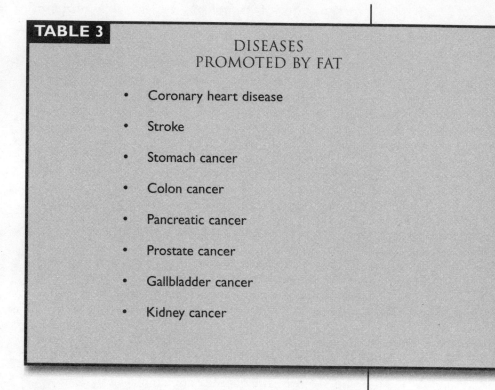

TABLE 3

DISEASES
PROMOTED BY FAT

- Coronary heart disease

- Stroke

- Stomach cancer

- Colon cancer

- Pancreatic cancer

- Prostate cancer

- Gallbladder cancer

- Kidney cancer

association between high dietary fat and prostate cancer need be provided than a look at the current rise in diseases related to dietary fats in countries like Japan and even our own 50th state, Hawaii.[77,78] An intake of 40% or more fat leads to this effect, but it can be reduced by dropping the amount of saturated fat.[79-81]

STICKS AND STONES

Fat and carbohydrates may even cause kidney stones. As Japanese diets have become more Westernized since World War II, the incidence of calcium oxalate kidney stones has increased. Oxalate, which is found in leafy green vegetables and protein, binds to calcium in urine when the saturation level goes up, due to dehydration or excess excretion of oxalate. Traditionally, stone formers have been told to avoid calcium and foods high in oxalate. But in a study done in Japan, researchers found that carbohydrates and fats were the more likely culprits.[82] Calcium binds to fatty acids in the bowel, indicating that fat consumption may be closely related to oxalate excretion and stone formation. Many types of carbohydrate-rich foods contain a considerable amount of oxalate. High blood sugar increases calcium absorption from the gut in addition to creating higher levels of insulin release.[83] So what's the answer to preventing kidney stones? Eat more protein instead of high glycemic, fat-laden carbohydrates.[84]

With all the publicity about men developing osteoporosis, you need to realize the calcium you

OILS & THEIR COMPOSITION OF FATS — TABLE 4

Oil	PU	MU	Total Unsat	Sat
Olive	9	77	86	14
Canola	36	58	94	6
Peanut	34	48	82	18
Corn	62	25	87	13
Soybean	61	24	85	15
Sunflower	77	14	91	9
Safflower	77	14	91	9
Palm	10	39	49	51
Coconut	5	9	14	86

feed your man from food can prevent kidney stones, while gulping down wads of calcium supplements can not only increase his risk of turning them into bedrock in his urinary system, but increase the chance he'll develop prostate cancer.[85] If you're interested in finding more ways to prevent kidney stones, read "The Kidney Stones Handbook" by Gail Savitz and Dr. Stephen Leslie. In another interesting twist, consuming grapefruit juice increased the risk of forming a kidney stone by 44%, while caffeinated coffee and wine reduced the risk.[86] Calcium can also interfere with his ability to break down and eliminate estrogen from his body, making too much 17 beta-estradiol and estrone available to his tissue.[87] Grapefruit juice can also alter the metabolism of many drugs, especially those for blood pressure and asthma. So play it on the safe side and have him take all his medication with water.[88,89]

Too much calcium can increase his risk for prostate cancer

THE PROTEIN CONTROVERSY

High-protein diets are being blamed for everything from osteoporosis to kidney failure. Dieticians warn us about too much protein in our diets, based upon the recommendations of the American Dietetic Association. However, their conclusions are based upon insulin dependent diabetics and people with compromised vascular problems, especially involving the kidneys. Only recently have dieticians begun to work with the healthy, as most of their work has been done in a hospital setting where bodies are understandably under physical stress.

When bodybuilders were put on either high (2.8gm of protein per 2.2 pounds of body weight) or moderately high (1.26 grams) protein diets, no effect was found on their kidney's ability to clear toxins.[90] Worries about making his body too acid are also unfounded, as sugar and starch cause more acidosis than does protein.[91] Remember, the more leaky and acidotic a cell becomes, the more rapidly premature aging sets in. It seems that arginine, an amino acid found in protein, actually protects his kidneys' sensitive filtering units.[92] By eating protein, he encourages his body to break down estrogen quicker, which makes more testosterone available to turn him into your favorite sand stud.

CARBOHYDRATE KRYPTONITE

Diets higher in protein than carbohydrates have been vilified in today's press, but a closer look at the mechanisms behind testosterone metabolism may prove that protein can defend him against impotency and heart disease caused by too much estrogen in his system. The synthesis and breakdown of estrogen involves enzymes, called cytochrome P-450, in liver and fat cells. A specific enzyme, estrogen-2-hydroxylase (E2OHase), converts estrone into a non-estrogenic metabolite that is excreted in urine. This enzyme is affected by drugs, body fat and the amount of protein in his diet.[93]

THE BIO-AVAILABILITY OF ESTRADIOL

Eating a protein-rich diet can help him get rid of estrogen

The metabolite, 2-OHE, binds to and prevents estrogen from taking over his testosterone receptors. Not so for 16-OHE, which attaches to the same receptor and increases the amount of available circulating estradiol. This can lead to impotency, heart disease and high blood pressure. Eating a protein-rich diet can increase the activity of his CP-450 enzymes, helping him to get rid of estrogen. When individuals were fed a diet of 44% protein and 35% carbohydrates, there was a profound affect on the activity in the 2-OHE pathway, favoring estrogen deactivation.[94] Even a low-fat diet can protect his tissue, shifting estradiol metabolism away from the

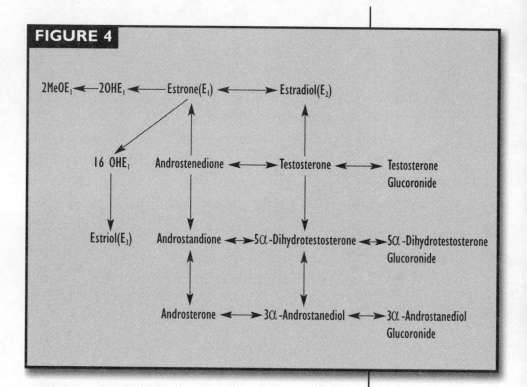

FIGURE 4

16-hydroxylation pathway and towards the estrogen de-activating 2-hydroxylation route.[95] It doesn't take a superman to understand that a diet composed of 40% protein, 25% fats and 35% low-glycemic carbohydrates can send him leaping into the air with a single bound!

EAT LIKE A GLADIATOR

Pythagoras (the athletic coach, not the philosopher) was the first to train gladiators and athletes on a meat diet supplemented with naturally-occurring carbohydrates, such as emmer wheat and barley. Like the French diet of today, his training table included beef, chicken, lamb, wild game, pork, fish, olives, wine and a considerable serving of vegetables.[38]

Modern researchers have proven the value of his training table when it comes to stimulating testosterone production. When researchers investigated the diets of strict vegetarians, they found testosterone levels were 18 percent lower and plummeted further after just one hour of exercise in athletes fed a vegetarian diet.[96,97]

Even the Brits reported that people who select foods with a low glycemic index – that is, foods that promote a steady, slow rise in blood sugar after a meal, rather than a rapid spike – have high enough levels of the good cholesterol, HDL, and triglycerides to lower their risk of heart disease by 29%.[98]

Scientists still aren't sure how dietary protein affects osteoporosis, even though protein is an important structural component of bone. In a study designed to evaluate the relationship between hip fractures and dietary protein intake, researchers found that eating protein, especially from animal sources, was actually beneficial in reducing the incidence of hip fractures.[99] Plus, eating fruits and vegetables high in potassium not only lowers his risk for prostate cancer but also protects his bones by reversing any urinary calcium loss.[100-102] So don't be afraid to serve him more lean protein. It could be just the leg he needs to stand on.

PHYTOESTROGENS: FRIEND OR FOE?

Phytoestrogens, which are contained in such foods as garlic and onions, help protect against impotency and heart disease by shifting the metabolism of estrogen to its inactive metabolites.[103]

Phytoestrogens can reduce cholesterol and help treat osteoporosis and even prostate enlargement in men.[104] Garlic and onions offer additional prostate protection while isoflavones, a component of beans and soy, had the beneficial effect of relaxing blood vessels.

The source of protein becomes important. Some phytoestrogens are high in protein. When you feed your man a diet chock-full of these foods, you are really serving him a protein-adequate diet. Just

TABLE 5	FOOD SOURCES OF PHYTOESTROGENS
Isoflavones	**Legumes**
	Soy beans, lentils, beans (haricot, broad, kidney, lima, chick peas)
	Products of beans
	Soy meal, soy grits, soy flour, tofu, soy milk
Lignans	**Whole grain cereals**
	Wheat, wheat germ, barley, hops, rye, rice, brans, oats
	Fruit, vegetables, seeds
	Cherries, apples, pears, stone fruits, linseed, sunflower seeds
	Carrots, fennel, onion, garlic
	Broccoli
	Vegetable oils including olive oil
	Alcoholic sources
	Beer from hops, bourbon from corn
Coumestans	**Bean sprouts**
	Alfalfa, soybean sprouts
	Fodder crops
	Clover

adding 25gm of soy protein a day can lower his cholesterol.[105] So if he's not getting enough protein, just make the difference up with foods rich in phytoestrogens.[106] The typical Asian diet includes forty milligrams of isoflavones per day, the equivalent of one serving of a soy food.[219] That's about 2 tablespoons of soy powder or 1/4 of the vacuum-packed tofu container. Soy also helps block his fat cells from converting androstenedione into estrogen.[107] As an additional benefit, it can also inhibit tyrosine kinase, an enzyme that helps prostate cancer cells to multiply.[108] But don't overdo it. Isoflavones, especially in the form of supplements, can turn off his thyroid and interfere with his hormone balance. It's a classic example of a little going a long way, just like your mother-in-law. So use common sense. Incorporate small amounts of low-glycemic phytoestrogens into his diet along with low-fat sources of protein for a healthy, gladiator lifestyle.

MEN AND ALCOHOL

Moderation is also the key to drinking. Moderate drinking (2 glasses of alcohol per day) can actually lower a man's chances of developing Type 2 diabetes.[109] However, any more than that can increase his metabolism of estrogen, which leads to impotency and brittle bones.[110] So don't let him be duped into believing the current press that wine is the way to beat heart disease, when a diet rich in fruits and vegetables can provide the same benefits.[62, 111, 112]

Alcohol can increase his metabolism of estrogen

Unfortunately, little effort has been made to provide non-alcoholic wines fortified with quercitin and resveratrol, the active ingredients believed to contribute to a healthy heart. In the United States, alcohol is the third-leading cause of premature death; its use and abuse results in more than 100,000 deaths annually and imposes more than $167 billion in economic damage on society. The rate of coronary heart disease may be relatively low, but deaths from alcohol-related digestive diseases and cancers, as well as unintentional injuries, are excessive, recently estimated at nearly 25% of all premature mortality. Official government policies in France, as in the United States, call for reductions in alcohol consumption. So if you want him to be your Iron Chef in bed, keep the alcohol down to one glass of beer or wine a day.

Caffeine can lower his sperm count

CAFFEINE: GROUNDS FOR CONCERN?

That cup of joltin' java turns out to be a lot safer than we thought in terms of cancer, but let him drink too much and he could sabotage his fertility and his efforts to lose weight. Dietary caffeine, specifically methylxanthine-containing beverages such as coffee and colas, have been blamed for bone loss and headaches. However, the risk of colon cancer was reduced in drinkers of 4 or more cups per day in over 10,000 people studied for 5 years.[113] Now that may seem like good news – but sprinkle some stress into the picture and things take on a different perspective. When male medical students were studied during exams, the combination of stress and caffeine significantly raised their blood pressure.[114] Even young healthy men had higher cortisol levels for more than two hours after drinking just 2 cups of coffee.[115] Remember, the longer cortisol stays up, the more resistant his body becomes to burning fat. In fact, drinking caffeine raises his blood sugar without stimulating insulin, which stops the release of glucagon. But that's not all. Drinking more than 4 cups a day of caffeinated coffee can turn off his ability to manufacture sperm, even if his testosterone levels are normal.[116] So if he consumes numerous cups a day, he may be making himself sterile and shutting down glucagon and his fat burning mechanism.[117]

LIQUID OXYGEN

Water is an overlooked nutrient. Within our bodies, it is the great transporter of nutrients, oxygen and waste products. It's a medium for chemical reactions. It cools and cushions our bodies, which are more than 50% water. In a way, we are mobile aquariums in which assorted organs slosh around like buoys in an ocean. To be well-hydrated the average man needs to consume nine cups of fluid per day in the form of soups, foods and (non-alcoholic) beverages. Solid food contributes about 4 cups of water with an additional 1 cup coming from oxidation in the body. It's been proven that consuming fluids in general and drinking water in particular cuts the risks of kidney stone disease, colon and urinary tract cancer, obesity, mitral valve prolapse and overall health.[118] Water is really liquid oxygen, made up of two parts hydrogen for every single oxygen molecule. Think of it as just another way of increasing the oxygen in his body. By drinking one liter of mineral water, he obtains his recommended dietary allowance of calcium (800 milligrams) without any absorption problems. So next time he's reaching for a cola, hand him some "Liquid Oxygen" instead.

IT'S AN EGG-XAGGERATION

The egg may not be the cholesterol-raising culprit it was once believed to be, especially as part of a low-saturated fat diet. It seems diets high in carbohydrates can impair his glucose tolerance and increase his triglyceride levels while reducing the good cholesterol in NIDDM individuals.[119] In fact, researchers are rethinking cholesterol's role in cardiovascular crimes. It seems people vary widely in their ability to metabolize cholesterol, and compensate for absorbed dietary cholesterol by decreasing the amount produced in the liver or by increasing the cholesterol excreted, along with bile, from the gallbladder. And if you want to protect his eyes, nothing can beat the humble egg yolk as the nutritional champ for levels of the carotenoids, lutein and zeaxanthin.[120]

THE CHOCOLATE DIET

No, I'm not recommending he consume a diet based on chocolate, but including some in his weekly Gladiator Diet Plan won't cause him any harm. It seems cocoa butter contains stearic acid, which can actually drop his cholesterol levels.[121] Although it is a highly saturated fat, it's melting point is above body temperature, making it less well absorbed. Even drinking a cup of hot cocoa can reduce the ability of his platelets to clump like girls at an 'N Sync concert, making it rival aspirin in effectiveness.[122] I recommend a California product by Scharffen Berger that contains 70% cocoa butter, but a Dove silky dark chocolate chunk or a Snickers bar will do in a pinch.

Chocolate can drop his cholesterol and protect him from a stroke

THE NON-NUTRIENT: FIBER

Dietary fiber helps protect him from exposure to active estrogens such as estrone and estradiol.[13] It seems having a regular bowel movement reduces the time in which estrogens can be reabsorbed from stool as it navigates the colon, which cuts down on the amount of circulating estrogen.[123] Fiber can also keep his blood sugar in check while helping him lose weight. Fiber can even protect him against cancer.[124] Try including fiber-rich foods in his diet, especially pears, apples and beans.

A PINCH OF SALT

Do you look at your man as if he were about to

drink battery acid any time he reaches for salt? Not to worry. We need salt to balance adrenal function. Our bodies are very complex, with the adrenals handling our steroid and salt/water balance. When a man becomes low in salt, his blood pressure drops and he feels light-headed. Salt attracts water into his plasma, which compensates for changes in his sympathetic nervous system. Calcium, magnesium and potassium, minerals found in natural sea salt, can lower his blood pressure while keeping fluid balance between his cells steady. Just think of his body as a complex stew pot...with all sorts of "flavors" bubbling away. While salt sensitivity is an inherited trait in African Americans, it has not been found in other races.[125] When healthy Chinese were given increasing doses of salt over a week, up to 4250 millimoles a day (that's about 8 tablespoons), there was no change in blood pressure.[126] A low salt diet can actually increase a man's blood glucose and insulin levels, especially if he has any form of hypertension.[127] So why has sodium been nailed for causing high blood pressure? Researchers now realize that iodine, nitrates, fluoride and other negative charged ions are the culprit in causing our "stew" to boil over. Just eliminating most processed foods, which contain these culprits, can put anyone in the normal range for sodium intake.

THE THYROID THEORY

Iodine was added to America's salt to prevent mental retardation from thyroid disease caused by iodine-deficient soil in areas such as the Ohio River Valley. However, iodine can cause significant changes in people with subclinical hypothyroidism, even in small doses.[128] In Japan, seaweed wraps, made from kelp which is high in iodine, caused marked hypothyroidism among those who ate them daily.[129] So using salt with iodine may be tipping the balance in his thyroid function.

If you taste table salt, it has a bitter flavor due to the chemicals that are added along with the iodine. In comparison, sea salt has a sweet taste. Try switching his salt to natural sea salt not treated with additional iodine. I bet you will find it takes very little to bring a new flavor balance to his food and his weight.

SWEET AS SUGAR

Much has been made about over-consumption of sugar in our country, but the use of fructose has increased steadily in the past two decades as a more natural substitute for sugar in soft drinks and yogurt. However, fructose raises cholesterol and causes more adverse effects on collagen, creating sagging skin and brittle bones.[130] When protein and fructose without any fat or carbohydrate were eaten together, the insulin response was the same as 3 tablespoons of corn syrup. Glucagon was suppressed, not stimulated, by the combination.[131] So he should eat fruit at least one hour before a meal, or add some fat along with the fruit or wait at least two hours after having any protein to keep his fat burning metabolism on high. Aspartame (Nutrasweet™) and other artificial sweeteners have been studied extensively in diabetics.[132] It seems bitter-tasting compounds, such as saccharin, sodium cyclamate, stevioside and acesulfame-K stimulate insulin release while sweet-tasting aspartame did not.[133] Taste buds are apparently critical in signaling the pancreas to release insulin. Although I could find no studies on sea salt and iodinated salt, I suspect there is a similar response.

THE GLADIATOR DIET

So, you ask, just how does a gladiator diet? The answer is...he doesn't. A gladiator understands how to maintain his optimum weight and testosterone levels by choosing foods that nourish his natural ability to remain fit and strong. But before I summarize everything, I want to be sure you understand that diets don't work...only changes in lifestyle can make a change in his weight, because stress and sleeplessness will counteract all the good eating habits he'll develop following this program. As you can understand from all I have said in the previous chapters, the regulation of body weight is a deceptively complex process, of which food selection is just one part. So how does he remember what to eat?

LIKE A TRUCKER'S MUDFLAP

If you've ever been behind a big rig on the road, you may have been amused or offended by the reclining female figure on a trucker's mudflap. However, if you keep that image in mind, neither of you will forget the percentage of low glycemic proteins/fats/carbohydrates he should average in his weekly diet:

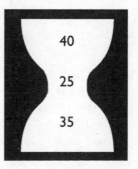

That's right. You want him to enjoy 40% of his foods as protein to encourage proper testosterone metabolism; keep his waistline below 34 by selecting 25% of his dict as fats and balance the remaining

35% of his food intake with low glycemic carbohydrates to supply his brain with enough glucose for
energy. 40/25/35 – that's the plan – and the shape!

You notice I said "average". It's unrealistic to
think he can manage this ratio at every meal or every
day. Aim for a weekly average. When he eats a meal
loaded with protein, make his next meal a little
lighter. By eating small meals frequently, he can
adjust his insulin response to the next meal, which
lets him draw or deposit into his carbohydrate
savings account, and that spells REFUND when he
consciously choses to eat a high glycemic carbohydrate or saturated fat.

How do you know if he is using the
recommended "shape" of The Gladiator Diet? It's
very simple. Just think of his plate as a clock. Fill the
portion between 12 and 5 o'clock with protein, the
section between 8 and 12 o'clock with low glycemic
carbohydrates, and the small space left in between
nicely holds a shotglass of fat. As low glycemic
carbohydrates contain more fiber, it's impossible to
"OD" on them unlike fat, so feel free to let him use
an extra "hour" on that clock.

HOW MANY MACHO MEALS DOES HE NEED?

It's very simple to figure out how many macho
meals he needs. The number of calories he burns at
rest is called his basal metabolic rate or BMR. To
calculate how many calories he needs just to sit still,
take his weight in pounds and multiply by 11. Divide
that figure by 350 and you have the number of
macho meals necessary just to keep him breathing.
Now add 350 calories for walking, jogging, fixing the
car or even just fidgeting and you have an idea of
how many calories are required just to maintain his
current weight. If you want him to lose weight,
simply deduct one macho meal and add 30 minutes

of moderate exercise a day to equal an approximate 700 calorie deficit. In just a week he will have lost one pound of fat. Keep it up and he can expect an average weight loss of five pounds the first month, and four pounds each month until he reaches his desired goals. The more muscle he has, the more fat burning cells are available to pulverize that lard, so don't get jealous when he drops the weight even faster.

Don't let him cheat, however, by eliminating two meals and not exercising or eating less than 4 meals a day. He'll just lose muscle and slow down his fat burning metabolism. Then the macho diet fairy in the pink tutu and motorcycle boots will come visit him and bring back all his fat plus more for good measure. That's a promise.

CHOOSING CARBOHYDRATES

Consider these high glycemic carbohydrates as "treats" to be used sparingly until he has achieved a normal BMI.

Apricots	Baked beans	Banana
Bread	Carrots	Cereals
Corn	Couscous	Cranberry sauce
Dates	Figs	Mango
Muffins	Noodles	Oat bran
Papaya	Parsnips	Pasta
Peas	Pickles, sweet	Potatoes
Raisins	Rice	Yams/sweet potatoes

This includes any form of these carbohydrates, especially fried or buttered versions, such as potato chips or popcorn. Remember, high glycemic carbohydrates, when treated with fat, react like 3 tablespoons of corn syrup in his body and prevent him from losing weight. If you want him to feel more energized, keep that stuff out of the house until he has achieved the following goals:

1. A waistline below 34 inches
2. Body fat percentage below 15%
   (10% is even better)
3. Body mass index below 25
4. A waist/hip ratio around 1.

In Chapter 8, I will show you how to calculate his body mass index and fat percentage. It is not weight that determines what is healthy for him, but these four factors. If he strives to achieve each one, he will have dropped his risk factors for fat-related diseases down to that of an 18-year-old gladiator...and who wouldn't want to be in those arms at night!

FIND THE FAT

His gallbladder needs 10gm of saturated fat at one time in order to empty completely.[134] That is precisely one tablespoon of unsalted butter. Meats and poultry, whether red or white, have varying degrees of saturated fat. Since these are "hidden" fats, that is, you don't see the fat, restrict his intake of red meat to twice a week. I have found it easiest to restrict saturated fat by using only 1 tablespoon of unsalted butter a day, and filling the rest of the fat allowance with mono-unsaturated fats in the form of olive oil. This has the additional advantage of cleaning up your kitchen cupboards, as you won't need to stock every form of polyunsaturated oil. Extra virgin olive oil contains the highest amount of mono-unsaturated fatty acids, with the percentage dropping with each subsequent pressing of the olives. However, for salads, I prefer the less flavorful "light" olive oil.

Don't confuse the name... there are no differences in calories here, only in the intensity of the flavor.

One tablespoon of butter seems skimpy unless you melt it in a very small container. Pyrex™ produces little glass containers that make a melted tablespoon look enormous, but shot glasses will do nicely. In addition, serving butter this way allows him to dip his low glycemic carbs into it, intensifying the flavor in his mouth while conserving fat grams. And don't forget to grind a few crystals of sea salt into that butter for a sweet, mouth-filling flavor.

If you've ever stood in front of the dairy section and worried about choosing the product with the least fat, you may be looking at the wrong ingredient. Excessive intake of milk and dairy products has been linked with prostate cancer in several countries.[85] Men need to watch their calcium intake if they want their prostate to remain healthy. Kosher yogurt, made with live cultures of acidophilus and no gelatin, offers a whopping 90% of his daily calcium needs in just one cup. Three and one-half ounces of gruyere cheese supplies him with 1011 milligrams of calcium, his limit, while cheddar and Monterey Jack provide a respectable 730 milligrams. Research has now shown that calcium binds with fat to form a "soap" which prevents his body from absorbing the fat in cheese and milk.[135] The downside? Calcium depletes the amount of zinc available to protect his prostate.[136]

Want him to have the torso of a Fabio? Cottage cheese may be the answer. A study of muscle strength showed the choice of cottage cheese over whey protein powder resulted in a 60% increase in leg, chest and shoulder strength.[137] California has enriched dairy products with calcium, making nonfat or 1% cottage cheese the best choice. So don't look just at the fat when choosing a dairy product. Read the label and select the product with the lowest percentages of both calcium and fat if you're looking to help him stay healthy while losing weight. If you find he just craves more saturated fat as he starts the

Calcium depletes zinc in his body

diet, try decreasing the frequency, not the amount, of saturated fat he eats in a day. Again, the French have proven variety in one's diet is the passbook to his weight-savings account.

PROTECTING WITH PROTEIN

There are several reasons to eat more protein than currently recommended, especially in light of its ability to direct testosterone metabolism. But too much protein can stress kidneys already affected by atherosclerotic disease. The ADA currently recommends a diet of no more than 15-20% protein. As I have already discussed, soy protein does not cause super filtration in the kidney, while helping to ward off cancer and regulate cholesterol. By adding an additional 15% protein in the form of soy, you can improve his cholesterol and help boost his testosterone levels. It's a hard fact!

It's easy to add soy to his diet with all the products available in today's supermarket. Try adding a tofu dog to a cup of soup, or sprinkle 1 scoop of the powder, which supplies 30 mg of isoflavones, into a hot bowl of Irish oatmeal. It's a natural for stir fry and blends up easily with Swiss Miss™ Diet Chocolate drink. Eat it as cheese or drink soy milk, which has only 16 mg of isoflavones. The possibilities are endless. Just remember that a little goes a long way and limit the amount of isoflavones to 190mg in a week. Learning to cook with soy can benefit your entire family.

FRUIT SMOOTHIES AND ENERGY BARS

It's tempting to suggest he have a fruit smoothie for breakfast to get energy on the run. However, when protein and fructose, the natural sugar in fruit, are combined without any fat, the response in the body is the same as if he ate several pieces of white bread or swallowed 3 tablespoons of corn syrup. So don't make the mistake of mixing a protein powder, such as whey or soy with water and fruit. Always make a protein drink with 1% milk. You'll keep his insulin and glucose levels under control and still have a tasty, nutritious treat. A liquid breakfast, however, doesn't balance his insulin response as well as a high fiber meal because it is absorbed at a much faster rate.[138] It's okay to use a liquid breakfast once a week, but don't make a habit of it or you'll find him hunting for those dangerous high sugar carbs before lunch.

When choosing fruits for his diet, concentrate on red/purple or dark blue fruits such as blueberries, blackberries, plums, huckleberries or dark red ones such as raspberries. Not only are they lower in fructose, but they also contain proanthocyanidins (PCA's), which can strengthen blood vessels such as capillaries and help prevent wrinkles, varicose veins or bruising.

Energy bars are another area of danger. Comprised of protein and carbohydrates, these bars use fructose, rice, barley or corn syrup as sweeteners and can build a "Buddha Belly" faster than he can chant a mantra! Look for new protein bars without corn syrup, such as "Source One" by MetRx, which are low in fructose, sucrose and fat.

EAT LIKE AN ELEPHANT

Nuts can help him lose weight

Putting away a few nuts may help him lose weight and protect his heart. Peanuts, almonds, macadamia, walnuts and cashews are excellent sources of mono-unsaturated fats, which can keep his arteries clean as a whistle. These calorie-dense snacks are versatile and easy to incorporate into meals. Just 5 ounces provides him with 50% of his daily Vitamin E and folic acid requirements, which lowers his risk of heart disease. Nuts also contain resveratrol, the compound in red wine that prevents the oxidation of LDL in his blood. Nuts won't add inches to his waistline if eaten in small quantities but they will go a long way in helping him feel satisfied with less saturated fat in his diet. Dry roasted, unsalted peanuts are ideal for snacking and cooking. A handful is about 2 ounces, so go ahead...toss them in a salad or stew.

THE SPICE IN LIFE

Nothing evokes memories of home cooking more than the smell of spices. Having traveled most of the "free inoculum world" or any place where you don't need a vaccination, I can instantly recall a country by its smell. From cardamom, anise and cloves in Denmark to cumin, cinnamon and turmeric in Morocco—each of these combinations gets my digestive juices flowing. Herbs de Provence, a combination of French lavender, basil, thyme, savory and fennel gives all foods a new zip. As an additional benefit, fennel seeds (also known as fenugreek) help to lower blood glucose.[139]

Sugar and spice make everything nice, especially when you use seasonings that contain chromium, a nutrient that helps maintain insulin sensitivity in his tissues. Scientists have discovered that spices such as cinnamon, tumeric, cloves, bay leaves and fennel seeds can triple insulin's ability to sweep glucose into his hungry cells.[140] No wonder that Greeks and Mexicans and the nomadic cultures of North Africa favor these spices in their cooking. And don't be afraid to add a little sugar to any of your recipes. Research has shown that sugar, when added to foods, has no additional effect on blood glucose levels than that of the sugar alone, and can prevent him from increasing his intake of fat and high glycemic carbohydrates.[141] Don't forget that salt is a spice. Sometimes just a few grinds of sea salt followed by a great cracked pepper is all you need to make a gourmet dinner. Experiment with the numerous spice combinations available at your local market. See Appendix A for sources of exotic and unusual spices. With just a little variety you can make cooking as adventuresome as a trip around the world.

TEA TIME

Tea is a medicinal drink in many cultures and a sign of friendship, as in Middle Eastern countries. Who isn't aware of the British penchant for afternoon tea or the symbolism of dumping it into Boston Harbor? Teas are really an infusion of hot water into the leaf of a plant in order to extract its essence. Some teas, such as green tea, have compounds that may protect against cancer. One cup of green or black tea has more antioxidant power than one-half cup of broccoli, carrots, spinach or strawberries. Just by drinking two cups a day, a man can lower his risk of aortic atherosclerosis by 46%, and by 69% with four cups a day.[142] With the wide variety of teas available, it's fun to make a different flavor every day. Mango and papaya teas contain enzymes that help digest fats and proteins. Brew tea by placing a jar of cold water in the sun (sun tea), leaving it out overnight, (moon tea) or by steeping it in hot water for 5 minutes. Decaffeinated teas are less acidic. I recommend Tejava, a mineral water tea made by Crystal Geyser Water Company and available in your grocery store.

Tea has compounds that may protect against cancer

THE HIDDEN SUGAR: CORN SYRUP

I was amazed when I seriously began to study food labels and discovered how many products contain corn syrup. Sold as "glucose" in England, corn syrup is in everything from tomato soup and juice to coffee cream substitutes. Due to the enormous excess of corn production in this country, it has become the number one sweetener in commercial products. And don't fall for rice or barley syrup as a substitute. They all have the same effect in his body. High fructose corn syrup depletes his body of vitamins and minerals and can lead to intracellular dehydration and aging. It's critical that you read the entire label on any product as you could inadvertently send his weight management program barreling off track by a simple mistake. But here's an interesting thought—if you stick to the fresh produce section instead of the aisles of the supermarket, you won't have to be so diligent.

MSG BY SO MANY NAMES

Steering clear of monosodium glutamate, or MSG, is about as easy as dodging death or taxes. Twenty million Americans are estimated to be sensitive to this food additive which is required by the FDA to be listed whenever it is an ingredient in foods. However, there is no law requiring manufacturers to declare components of any ingredient. Additives such as hydrolyzed vegetable protein (HVP), autolyzed yeast or yeast extract, and sodium and calcium caseinate all contain potentially threatening amounts of MSG, making up between 8 to 40 percent of HVP. Again, as it is used mainly as a preservative and flavor enhancing agent, that's another good reason to stay in the produce section.

PORTIONS: SIZE **DOES** MATTER

The issue of portion control is a hot one in weight management. If you're hungry, you will eat bigger portions because your stomach is slow to tell your brain that it's full and had enough. Remember, hormones in your gut are responsible for e-mailing your brain to tell your hand to put the fork down.

The greatest reason for lack of portion control is the hormonal imbalance created by delayed gastric emptying. But in a study done with men of normal weight, just presenting them with larger portions resulted in their consuming twice the amount of food they normally ate. It seems those super-sized portions encourage overeating in anyone![143] Afraid he'll think you're serving him a portion fit for a sparrow instead of a vulture? Use smaller plates. (Men are so easy to fool!)

You can even impress him with how much money you're saving by shopping like a gladiator. By starting at the fresh produce and dairy sections, you'll make fewer trips down aisles filled with shelf-stable high glycemic carbohydrates, and fewer stops at the bakery. Experiment with the wide range of available fresh fish and select only lean red meat for his twice-weekly indulgence. The amount of food you'll buy will drop as you realize he can do with smaller portions of meat and more vegetables and fruit. Remember, each bite of food gives you a new opportunity to revitalize and energize his metabolism, so choose wisely!

PRINCIPLES OF THE GLADIATOR DIET

Consume a diet averaging:

- 40% protein to encourage proper testosterone metabolism

- 25% fat (15% mono-unsaturated fats and 10% saturated)

- 35% low glycemic carbohydrates

- Eat five to six macho meals a day beginning with breakfast

- Exercise 30 minutes a day

- Eat one serving of soy a day

- Begin every meal with a small snack of protein

- Use non-iodinated sea salt

- Enjoy five ounces of nuts a week

- Drink one glass of wine a day

- Drink four eight-ounce glasses of water a day, preferably mineral water

- Reduce caffeine

- Eat low fat, low-calcium dairy products in limited amounts

- Use one tablespoon of unsalted butter daily

- Never consume fruit and proteins together without some fat

- If you eat a high glycemic carbohydrate, don't add fat

CHAPTER 4
A Man, A Can
and a 7 Day Plan

There's truth to the rumor the best way to a man's heart is through his stomach, especially if you serve him a balanced, low glycemic meal. However, you don't have to become a kitchen slave in order to provide your warrior with the right foods to enhance his testosterone. It's as easy as opening a can.

To start, you need to make two copies of Table 6 in this chapter. Keep one in your purse and post the other on your refrigerator (in case anyone else in the family should feel moved to do the shopping for you!). This will insure you have a workable list of allowable ingredients, which can be turned into anything from a simple nosh to a gourmet meal. Next, you need to clean out your cupboards and eliminate any canned goods that are based on the high glycemic list on page 43. Fill the space instead with soups that don't contain high fructose corn syrup, maltodextrin, MSG or large amounts of potatoes or corn. Add cans of kidney, garbanzo (chick peas) and white navy beans to your stockpile. Fat free chicken and white meat tuna in water look great next to cans of tomatoes and fat free chicken broth. Throw in some sugar-free jello flavors, Swiss Miss™ Diet Chocolate mix and you're almost done.

Next, get rid of polyunsaturated oils and purchase extra-virgin olive oil, canola and peanut oil for daily use. If you are feeling adventuresome, select nut oils, such as walnut or almond for additional flavor. Oil misters are available, which can let you spray your selected oil on any surface. Finally, clear some space for various vinegars, such as balsamic, red wine, apple cider, rice wine or white vinegar, and your cupboards will be clean and organized.

Spices are essential and should be fresh. That means the container of cumin you bought six months ago is toast! Purchase the smallest amount of any spice to be certain you use it within three months if you want to enjoy the maximum fragrance and flavor these condiments supply.

Don't forget the salt. I keep one package of kosher salt by the stove, and fill a salt grinder with natural non-iodinated sea salt. Finally, invest in a pepper mill and experience the aroma and mouth-filling flavor of freshly ground pepper. It can turn any dish into a prize winner.

The refrigerator needs a once over. Eliminate margarines and purchase unsalted (sweet cream) butter. As dairy products tend to have more hormones in them than Mark McGuire, I would recommend certified organic products whenever possible. Vitamin D is lost when fat is removed from dairy, so choose low fat but not non-fat products. Stock up on omega-3 fortified eggs and keep lean, pork loin (Canadian bacon) in your refrigerator for breakfast or anytime.

Cereals and breads are best if made from spelt or whole wheat berries. Remember, a product must say stone ground whole wheat to qualify as a moderate glycemic grain. Whole wheat pitas are another good product, as they can be turned into wraps, pizza bases and great sandwiches without fear of sending anyone's blood sugar to the top of Crystal Mountain.

THE GLADIATOR DIET
RECOMMENDED FOOD LIST

TABLE 6

PROTEINS	CARBOHYDRATES (MODERATE GLYCEMIC)	CARBOHYDRATES (LOW GLYCEMIC)
turkey breast	stone ground whole wheat	asparagus
lean ground turkey	spelt breads	broccoli
chicken breast	spelt/kamut cereal	green beans
lean ground chicken	steel cut oatmeal	spinach
tuna in water	whole wheat pita bread	tomato
98% fat free chicken in water	barley	peppers
salmon	wild rice	zucchini
swordfish	apple	cucumber
shrimp	blueberries	celery
crab	blackberries	brussels sprouts
lobster	raspberries	lettuce
orange roughy	kidney beans	onions
sole	garbanzo beans	cabbage
pork loin	navy beans	cauliflower
lean ham/Canadian bacon	low-fat yogurt	cherries
top sirloin steak	squash	dried apricots
top round steak	farro pasta/whole wheat pasta	pears
lean ground beef	All-bran cereal	plum
buffalo	grapes	kiwi
eggs	sweet potato	nuts
low-fat cottage cheese	yam	bean thread noodles

Now that you have your list, let me show you how easy it is to provide quality nutrition in twenty minutes or less.

DAY 1

Breakfast:
Mix one scoop whey protein powder with one cup low-fat yogurt, fresh or frozen berries, crushed ice and blend at high speed for 45 seconds.
Midmorning:
apple with string cheese sticks
Lunch:
Four bean soup with ham, one slice stone ground whole wheat bread
Midafternoon:
individual container low-fat cottage cheese, two slices of fresh turkey
Dinner:
Sear roasted salmon, steamed green beans with unsalted butter, microwaved yam
Before 8pm:
Dove dark chocolate bar

DAY 2

Breakfast:
Two poached eggs with two slices Canadian bacon
Midmorning:
Microwaveable lentil soup
Lunch:
Whole wheat pita sandwich with tuna, tomatoes, cucumbers
Midafternoon:
grapes and peanuts
Dinner:
Grilled top sirloin steak, wild rice, steamed broccoli with unsalted butter
Before 8pm:
Sugar free jello with berries, fresh whipped cream flavored with left - over coffee

DAY 3

Breakfast:
Oat bran cereal with low fat or soy milk
Midmorning:
dried apricots, walnuts
Lunch:
Vegetarian chili and one slice stone ground whole wheat bread
Midafternoon:
fruit cup and cottage cheese
Dinner:
Seasoned grilled chicken breast , golden acorn squash with 1 tablespoon unsalted butter, broccoli topped with one slice melted gruyere cheese
Before 8 pm:
One glass of red wine

DAY 4

Breakfast:
Peanut butter smoothie made with natural nutty peanut butter and yogurt
Midmorning:
apple dipped in Swiss Miss™ Diet Chocolate Mix, lean deli ham slices
Lunch:
Mandarin orange chicken salad
Midafternoon:
microwaveable minestrone soup
Dinner:
Pork loin, summer squash, yam with 1 tablespoon unsalted butter
Before 8pm:
Waldorf salad (strawberries, grapes, apples, celery, walnuts)

DAY 5

Breakfast:
Scrambled eggs with lox, stone ground whole wheat bread

Midmorning:
Turkey slices rolled with provolone cheese slices, dill pickle

Lunch:
Crab salad with radishes, tomatoes, olives, bib lettuce, full fat mayonnaise diluted with canned crab juice

Midafternoon:
cottage cheese and fruit

Dinner:
Marinated flank steak, zuccini in marinara sauce, stone ground bread with 1 tablespoon unsalted butter

Before 8pm:
one glass red wine

DAY 6

Breakfast:
Steel cut Irish oatmeal with soy powder or milk, almonds

Midmorning:
nuts, yogurt

Lunch:
Buffalo mozzarella, tomatoes, basil and tuna salad

Midafternoon:
Oat bran cereal, low fat milk

Dinner:
Shrimp kabobs, grilled vegetables, wild rice with 1 tablespoon unsalted butter

Before 8pm:
chocolate shake with whey protein powder

DAY 7

Breakfast:
Spelt raisin bread with 1 tablespoon unsalted butter, soft boiled egg and lean ham

Midmorning:
yogurt with cantaloupe

Lunch:
Pita sandwich with chicken, onions, tomato, cucumber, Swiss cheese, lettuce

Midafternoon:
Salad made from lettuce, cucumbers, fennel, tomatoes, goat cheese

Dinner:
Chicken stir fry on bean thread noodles, broccoli, peppers, bean shoots, water chestnuts, tofu

Before 8pm:
Grilled portabello mushroom pizza

DON'T FRY FOR ME

Fast food needn't be a trap if your gladiator sticks to these entrees which are reasonably low in fat and high in fiber and water – key elements which make them denser and more filling. Avoid fried foods, which can pack on pounds faster than Elvis in the 70's.

Now that you understand how simple it is to eat like a gladiator, let me show you recipes guaranteed to turn any man into your warrior prince. Just remember that women and kids need 250 calorie versus 350 calorie meals. All you need do at each meal is add one quarter additional protein serving to another portion of low glycemic vegetables for your macho man to feel satisfied. And if you're interested in more delicious ways to cook for your entire family, "The Menopause Diet Mini Meal Cookbook" contains over 125 recipes that will cut cravings and keep your family slim and healthy. You can find out how to order this book in Appendix A.

TABLE 7	FAST FOOD CHOICES				
BRAND	CALORIES	% FAT CALORIES	PROTEIN(g)	CARBS (g)	FAT (g)
Taco Bell Grilled Chicken Burrito	390	30	19	49	13
Wendy's Grilled Chicken Sandwich	310	23	27	35	8
Subway Veggie Delite Sandwich	232	11	9	43	3
Subway Turkey Breast Sandwich	282	12	17	45	4
McDonald's Grilled Chicken Deluxe Plain	300	15	27	38	5
Carl's Junior BBQ Chicken Sandwich	280	11	25	37	3

NAKED SWEET POTATOES

Serves 4
per portion
Calories: 85
Protein: 1g
Carbs: 15g
Fat: 2g
Sat: 1g

Sweet potatoes are a great source of vitamins A and C and can be prepared in this simple, quick manner, which leaves them moist and naturally sweet.

3 (1/2 pound) dark-fleshed sweet potatoes
nonstick cooking spray
2 teaspoons olive oil
sea salt
2 cloves minced garlic
2 tablespoons finely minced sage
juice of 1/2 lime

Cut potatoes lengthwise into 1/2-inch-thick slices. Arrange slices in single layer on a baking sheet lightly sprayed with cooking spray. Brush the wedges with oil and sprinkle with coarse salt to taste and garlic.

Bake at 375 degrees until potatoes are fork tender, about 25 minutes. Sprinkle with sage and drizzle with lime juice.

CHILLY VIRGIN

Serves 2
per serving
Calories: 98
Protein: 4g
Carbs: 21g
Fat: 1g
Sat: 0g

Here's a new take on the "Virgin Mary". It's a great way to use cherry tomatoes in season and the frozen tomatoes won't dilute the sweet spicy taste.

2 pounds cherry tomatoes
freshly grated horseradish to taste
2 tablespoons freshly squeezed lime juice
Tabasco to taste

Freeze cherry tomatoes the night before using.

To make the Chilly Virgin drink, put all the ingredients except Tabasco into the blender. Garnish with celery stalks and an unfrozen cherry tomato.

PECOS BILL'S POBLANO AND TOMATO SALAD

This salad is a great way to use another member of the pepper family, poblano chili peppers, which are found in most grocery stores. Their heat can vary, so remove the seeds and ribs if you like it cool!

Serves 4
per serving
Calories: 67
Protein: 4g
Carbs: 10g
Fat: 2g
Sat: 1g

4 poblano chili peppers
2 tomatoes, diced
1/2 cup thinly sliced red onion
2 cloves garlic, minced
1 teaspoon dried Mexican oregano
3 tablespoons chopped cilantro
3 tablespoons lime juice
1/2 teaspoon sea salt
butter leaf lettuce
1/4 cup crumbled cotija cheese
wedges of lime dipped in chili powder, for garnish

Roast chiles on a rack over a open flame or under a broiler until charred on all sides. Place in a brown paper bag and close. Let chiles stand 15 minutes to sweat, then peel. Cut in half and remove seeds and ribs. Cut chiles lengthwise into strips.

Toss chiles with tomatoes, onion, garlic, oregano, cilantro, lime juice and salt. Cover and let rest 30 minutes. Line platter or serving plate with butter lettuce. Spoon salad atop greens and sprinkle with cheese. Garnish with lime wedges.

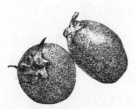

FETA AND TOMATO SPREAD

Serves 4
per serving
(including Pita)
Calories: 130
Protein: 5g
Carbs: 6g
Fat: 10g
Sat: 5g

This dish makes a simple hor d'oeuvre that is delicious served with mini whole wheat pita toasts.

4 ounces feta (French is less salty than Greek)
2 plum tomatoes
1 tablespoon extra-virgin olive oil
2 teaspoons finely chopped fresh oregano leaves
    or 1 teaspoon dried oregano, crumbled
freshly ground black pepper
whole wheat pita, small, cut into 4 pieces and toasted

Preheat broiler.
Crumble feta and spread evenly in a shallow flameproof baking dish (roughly 1-inch deep).
Thinly slice tomatoes crosswise and arrange, overlapping if necessary, on feta. Drizzle oil (or spray oil from a mister) over tomatoes and sprinkle with oregano and pepper. Broil mixture 2 to 3 inches from heat until cheese is bubbling, 5 to 8 minutes.
Serve spread with pita toasts.

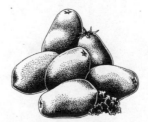

MINTED ZUCCHINI SALAD

If you find mysterious amounts of zucchini appearing on your doorstep at night, you probably have neighbors playing "zucchini fairy" with their overabundant crops. Here's a great recipe that's a snap to make anytime you find a "bumper crop" of these delicious squashes.

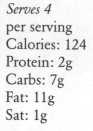

Serves 4
per serving
Calories: 124
Protein: 2g
Carbs: 7g
Fat: 11g
Sat: 1g

1 tomato
1 1/2 tablespoons fresh lemon juice
3 tablespoons extra-virgin olive oil
1/3 cup packed fresh mint leaves
1/4 cup packed fresh flat-leafed parsley leaves
3 medium zucchini (about 1 pound)

Cut tomato into 1/4-inch dice and transfer to a small bowl. In another small bowl whisk together lemon juice, oil, and salt and pepper to taste.

In a food processor finely chop mint and parsley. Replace chopping blade with shredding disk and shred zucchini over herbs. Transfer mixture to a large bowl. Drizzle three fourths vinaigrette over zucchini and toss with salt and pepper to taste. Pour off any juices from diced tomato and toss tomato with remaining vinaigrette and salt and pepper to taste.

Divide zucchini salad among 4 plates, mounding it, and make an indentation in center of each mound.

Fill indentations with tomatoes and garnish with mint.

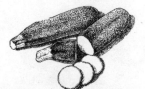

JAVELIN SALAD

Serves 4
per serving
Calories: 210
Protein: 20g
Carbs: 7g
Fat: 7g
Sat: 1g

This is a terrific way to incorporate nuts into a meal, which can spearhead his fight against heart disease. It even goes well accompanied by fresh fruit.

12 ounces green beans, trimmed, halved crosswise
2 cups shredded roasted chicken breast meat (about
    3 halves or 3 5-ounce cans white chicken in water)
1 cup thinly sliced red onion
5 tablespoons chopped fresh cilantro
2 teaspoons curry powder
1/3 cup plain nonfat yogurt
1 tablespoon mayonnaise
1 tablespoon fresh lime juice
2 teaspoons sliced almonds, toasted

Cook beans in pot of boiling salted water until crisp-tender, about 5 minutes. Rinse under cold water. Drain well. Transfer beans to large bowl. Add chicken, onion and 4 tablespoons cilantro.

Stir curry powder in small skillet over medium heat until aromatic, about 30 seconds. (Much longer and you will cough!) Transfer to small bowl. Whisk in yogurt, mayonnaise and lime juice. Add dressing to chicken mixture; toss to coat. Season to taste with salt and pepper. Sprinkle with almonds and remaining 1 tablespoon cilantro. Cover and chill or serve immediately.

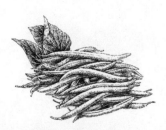

THE TERMINATOR SALAD

Chick peas, or garbanzo beans, are great for keeping blood sugar under control, which can terminate his cravings for junk food. This salad is tasty on its own or used as a stuffing for pita halves.

Serves 4
per serving
Calories: 265
Protein: 20g
Carbs: 36g
Fat: 5g
Sat: 1g

1/4 cup plain nonfat yogurt
3 tablespoons low-fat mayonnaise
1 1/2 tablespoons Dijon mustard
1 6-ounce can solid white tuna in spring water, drained
2 tablespoons fresh lemon juice
1 15– to 16–ounce can chickpeas (garbanzo beans), rinsed, drained
1 cup chopped sweet onion
1 cup chopped celery
1 cup cherry tomatoes, halved
1/2 cup chopped fresh Italian parsley

Whisk yogurt, mayonnaise, mustard and lemon peel in small bowl to blend.

Toss tuna with lemon juice in large bowl. Add chickpeas, onion, celery, tomatoes, parsley and yogurt dressing to bowl. Toss to blend. Season salad to taste with salt and pepper. (Can be made 6 hours ahead. Cover and chill.)

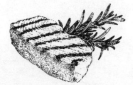

GREEK ADONIS CHICKEN SALAD

Serves 4
per serving
Calories: 234
Protein: 19g
Carbs: 21g
Fat: 7g
Sat: 2g

Here's another recipe that fits well in a pita pocket and will make your man into an Adonis in no time. Just line the pita with a lettuce leaf to prevent it from getting soggy before lunch or a snack.

2 cups cooked chicken breast (8 ounces or
    2 5-ounce cans white chicken in water)
1/2 diced, seeded, peeled cucumber
1/4 cup (1 ounce) crumbled feta cheese
1/8 cup chopped fresh parsley
1 tablespoon sliced, pitted kalamata olives
1/2 cup plain nonfat yogurt
1 tablespoon mayonnaise
1 tablespoon dried oregano
2 garlic cloves, minced
2 (6-inch) pitas, each cut in half
4 Boston lettuce leaves

Combine first 5 ingredients in large bowl. Combine yogurt, mayonnaise, oregano, and garlic in a small bowl. Pour over chicken mixture; toss well. Cover and chill 2 hours.

Line each pita half with a lettuce leaf, and fill with 1/2 cup chicken salad.

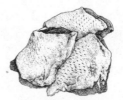

GRILLED CHICKEN AND PEAR SALAD

You can use any acceptable fruit to combine with simple, grilled chicken to have a wonderful meal ready in a flash. I use raspberries, pears and grapes but apples and kiwi give it a definite New Zealand flair.

Serves 4
per serving
Calories: 160
Protein: 5g
Carbs: 22g
Fat: 6g
Sat: 1g

4 skinless, boneless chicken breast halves
4 tablespoons fresh lime juice
2 tablespoons fresh chopped thyme or 2 teaspoons dried
1 teaspoon plus 1 tablespoon extra-virgin olive oil
sea salt, pepper
1 small garlic clove, minced
5 pears, thinly sliced
    (about 2 cups or 1 can of pears in light syrup)
1 cup grapes
6 cups mixed salad greens (spinach, red leaf lettuce,
    romaine...or your favorite bagged mixture)
1 tablespoon almond slices, toasted
1/2 cup fresh raspberries

Place chicken in a large plastic bag. Sprinkle with 1 tablespoon lime juice, 1 tablespoon thyrme and 1 teaspoon extra-virgin olive oil. Season with salt and pepper. Seal bag and massage ingredients into the chicken. Refrigerate 1 to 4 hours.

Prepare a grill or heat large nonstick skillet over medium-high heat. Grill or saute chicken until golden brown and just cooked through, about 5 minutes per side. Cool. Cut across the grain in thin diagonal slices.

Whisk 3 tablespoons lime juice, 1 tablespoon thyme, 1 tablespoon oil and garlic in large bowl. Season with salt and pepper. Place pear slices in small bowl; add 1 tablespoon dressing and toss to coat. Add salad greens to remaining dressing; toss to coat. Divide salad greens equally among 4 plates. Arrange sliced chicken atop each. Top with pears. Sprinkle with almonds. Garnish with raspberries.

BODICE RIPPER SMOOTHIES

Serves 1
per serving
without fruit
Calories: 206
Protein: 40g
Carbs: 14g
Fat: 5g
Sat: 2g

with fruit
Calories: 220
Protein: 40g
Carbs: 17g
Fat: 5g
Sat: 3g

It's easy to come up with variations on this drink that are high in protein, which can keep any man's testosterone in a bodice-ripping frenzy. I like to use low-fat vanilla yogurt for extra flavor and sweetness.

Basic recipe:
1/4 cup low-fat vanilla yogurt
3/4 cup chilled 2% fat milk
1 scoop whey protein powder (or 1 scoop soy powder)
pinch of sea salt
ice cubes

Add any of the following:
2 tablespoons applesauce
2 tablespoons berries
    raspberries
    blackberries
    boysenberries
    blueberries
1 tablespoon nutty natural peanut butter with
    1 package Swiss Miss™ Diet Chocolate Mix
1 cup pear slices in light syrup
1 tablespoon sliced almonds

COWBOY BEANS

During roundup, cowboys saved any extra coffee for use in cooking, as water was scarce. You can use leftover coffee or coffee powder in this adaptation. He'll be singing your praises with this dish.

Serves 4
per serving
Calories: 199
Protein: 6g
Carbs: 28g
Fat: 7g
Sat: 1g

2 tablespoons extra-virgin olive oil
1 onion, chopped
1 green bell pepper, chopped
2 tablespoons chopped garlic
2 bay leaves
2 1/2 tablespoons chili powder
1/2 tablespoon dried oregano
1 teaspoon ground cumin
1 1/2 cups water
1 8-ounce can tomato sauce
1 tablespoon instant coffee powder or 1 cup
   brewed coffee
3 15-ounce to 16-ounce cans pinto beans,
   rinsed and drained

Heat oil in heavy, large saucepan over medium heat. Add onion, green pepper, garlic and bay leaves. Saute until vegetables are almost tender, about 10 minutes. Add chili powder, oregano and cumin and saute 5 minutes. Mix in water, tomato sauce, and coffee powder. Add beans. Bring to boil. Reduce heat to medium-low; simmer until mixture thickens, stirring occasionally, about 45 minutes. Season with salt and pepper. (Can be made 1 day ahead. Cover and chill. Before serving, rewarm over low heat, stirring frequently.)

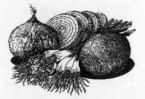

PORTABELLA PIZZAS

Serves 4
per serving
Calories: 141
Protein: 5g
Carbs: 22g
Fat: 5g
Sat: 1g

A great way to serve portabella mushrooms is to stuff them, but they're not very deep. Instead, they make a great "pizza crust". Be sure to remove the "gills" with a teaspoon so you have enough room for your favorite, delicious fillings.

Preparing the caps:

After removing the gills, spray the caps with olive oil and sear them in a hot pan for 5 minutes or grill them.

Fillings:

1 1/2 tablespoons extra-virgin olive oil
1 sprig rosemary
1 minced garlic clove
1 15-ounce to 16-ounce can white beans
    (navy beans or small white beans), drained
3/4 cup seeded and diced tomatoes

Heat olive oil in a medium skillet over high heat and add a lightly crushed 4-inch sprig of rosemary and heat for few minutes to release its aroma. Add the minced garlic and cook until tender. Add the white beans and cook for another 5 minutes. Add the tomatoes and toss to combine. Season with salt and pepper. Discard the rosemary and divide among four potabella caps.

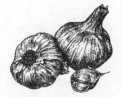

WHITE BEANS WITH OLIVE OIL, TOMATOES AND SAGE

2 tablespoons extra-virgin olive oil
1/4 cup coarsely chopped fresh sage
2 tablespoons coarsely chopped garlic
8 medium tomatoes (about 2 pounds or 1 can
   of crushed tomatoes)
1 15-ounce to 16-ounce can of white, Northern beans

Serves 4
per serving
Calories: 151
Protein: 5g
Carbs: 20g
Fat: 7g
Sat: 1g

Heat oil in heavy large saucepan over medium heat. Add chopped sage and chopped garlic and saute until garlic is golden, about 2 minutes. Add tomatoes and cook until sauce thickens slightly, about 10 minutes. Add beans to saucepan. Season to taste with salt and pepper. Cook until heated through, about 5 minutes.

ORANGES WITH CINNAMON, CAYENNE AND CHOCOLATE

This dish is packed with spices that balance blood sugar, improve your cholesterol and help with digestion...so what's not to love?

Serves 4
per serving
Calories: 79
Protein: 1g
Carbs: 17g
Fat: 1g
Sat: 1g

4 medium navel oranges
1/4 teaspoon cinnamon
Pinch of cayenne pepper
1/2 ounce Mexican chocolate, or semisweet
   chocolate, finely shaved

Peel the oranges removing the bitter white pitch. Working over a bowl, cut in between the membranes to release the orange sections. Squeeze the juice from the membranes into the bowl. Stir in the cinnamon and cayenne. Cover and refrigerate until chilled, for up to 2 hours.
Spoon the oranges and juice into individual bowls, sprinkle the shaved chocolate on top and serve.

SAUTEED KALE WITH SESAME SEEDS

Serves 4
per serving
Calories: 79
Protein: 2g
Carbs: 4g
Fat: 7g
Sat: 1g

1 1/2 cups water
1 bunch kale (about 1 pound), stems trimmed,
    leaves chopped
1 tablespoon extra-virgin olive oil
2 garlic cloves, minced
1/2 teaspoon dried, crushed red pepper
2 teaspoons oriental sesame oil
2 teaspoons sesame seeds, toasted

Bring 1 1/2 cups water to boil in heavy large Dutch over high heat. Add kale cover and boil until almost tender, stirring occasionally, about 4 minutes. Uncover, cook until liquid evaporates, about 3 minutes. (Can be made 4 hours ahead. Cover; let stand at room temperature.)

Heat olive oil in heavy large skillet over medium heat. Add garlic and dried red pepper flakes; saute 1 minute. Add kale; saute until heated through, about 3 minutes. Transfer to bowl. Drizzle with sesame oil and toss to coat. Season with salt and pepper. Top with sesame seeds.

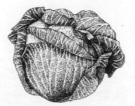

GREEN BEANS WITH WALNUTS AND WALNUT OIL

Here is a stylish treatment for green beans. I prefer the tiny, french haricots vert, but Kentucky Blue Lake beans work well, if you don't overcook them.

1 pound green beans, trimmed
1 tablespoon unsalted butter
2 teaspoons walnut oil
1/2 cup chopped walnuts (about 2 ounces), toasted
1 tablespoon minced fresh parsley

Cook beans in large pot of boiling sea salted water until just tender, about 5 minutes. Drain. Rinse beans with cold water and drain. (Can be prepared 6 hours ahead. Let stand at room temperature.)

Melt butter with oil in heavy large skillet over moderate heat. Add beans and toss until heated through, about 4 minutes. Season with sea salt and pepper. Add walnuts and parsley and toss. Transfer to bowl and serve.

Serves 4
per serving
Calories: 153
Protein: 5g
Carbs: 5g
Fat: 14g
Sat: 3g

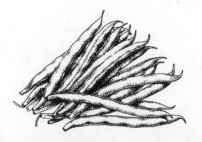

BUTTERNUT SQUASH WITH ONIONS AND PECANS

Serves 4
per serving
Calories: 165
Protein: 2g
Carbs: 9g
Fat: 15g
Sat: 4g

Here's another delectable way to incorporate nuts into healthy recipes.

1 tablespoon unsalted butter
1 medium white onion, finely chopped
1-1 1/2 pounds butternut squash, peeled, seeded,
    cut into 1/2-inch cubes (about 3 cups)
1/2 cup coarsely chopped pecans (about 2 ounces),
    toasted
1 tablespoon minced fresh parsley

Melt butter in heavy large skillet over low heat. Add onion and saute until very tender, about 15 minutes. Add squash and toss to coat. Cover and cook until squash is tender but still holds its shape, stirring frequently, about 15 minutes. Season with sea salt and pepper. (Can be prepared 4 hours ahead. Let stand at room temperature. Rewarm over medium heat before proceeding to the next step.) Stir in half of pecans and half of parsley. Transfer to bowl. Sprinkle with remaining pecans and parsley and serve.

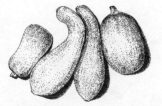

FENNEL TSATSIKI

This is a different take on the Greek dish, tsatsiki, which usually contains cucumbers. It's a great accompaniment to any grilled fish or lamb dish.

1 medium fennel bulb with fronds
    (sometimes called anise; about 3/4 pound)
1 teaspoon fennel seeds
2 garlic cloves
1 lemon
2 cups plain non-fat yogurt (16 ounces)
1 1/2 teaspoons sea salt

Trim fennel stalks flush with bulb, reserving fronds and discarding stalks, and trim any discolored outer layers. Halbe bulb lengthwise and discard core. Finely chop fronds and bulb. In a dry small skillet toast fennel seeds over moderate heat, shaking skillet, until fragrant and a shade darker. In an electric coffee/spice grinder, grind seeds. Mince garlic and squeeze lemon juice from lemon.

In a large bowl stir together chopped fennel, ground fennel seeds, garlic, yogurt, salt, and lemon juice to taste. May be made 3 days ahead and chilled, covered.

Makes 3 cups
per 4 ounce serving
Calories: 56
Protein: 4g
Carbs: 10g
Fat: 0g
Sat: 0g

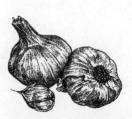

SAUTEED SPINACH CHIFFONADE WITH SHALLOTS

Serves 2
per serving
Calories: 109
Protein: 6g
Carbs: 8g
Fat: 8g
Sat: 1g

3/4 pound spinach (about 1 bunch)
2 large shallots, minced
1 tablespoon extra-virgin olive oil

Discard stems from spinach and wash thoroughly and drain. Working in batches, stack leaves on top of one another and cut into 1/2-inch-wide strips.

In a large heavy skillet cook shallots in oil over moderate heat, stirring, until softened. Add spinach and salt and pepper to taste and saute over moderately high heat, stirring, until wilted and tender, about 3 minutes.

GREEK SALAD WITH TUNA

Serves 4
per serving
Calories: 201
Protein: 17g
Carbs: 5g
Fat: 13g
Sat: 5g

This is so simple, but makes a great starter. It can also be used in a pita pocket for a delicious sandwich.

1/2 English seedless cucumber
1/2 pound cherry tomatoes
1/3 cup Kalamata olives
3 ounces feta
6-ounce can tuna in olive oil

Halve cucumber lengthwise and cut crosswise into 1/4-inch-thick pieces. Quarter tomatoes. Pit and quarter olives. Cut feta into 1/4-inch dice. In a bowl toss together cucumber, tomatoes, olives, feta, tuna with oil from can, and salt and pepper to taste, keeping tuna in large chunks.

CREAMY ZUCCHINI SOUP

Nutmeg adds a terrific flavor to this delicious soup, especially if you use a fresh seed. Simply grate it over the soup during the final heating for an aroma fit for a god!

1 1/2 pounds zucchini, cut into 1/2-inch pieces
1 1/2 cups canned low-salt, reduced fat chicken broth
1/4 cup whipping cream
1/4 teaspoon fresh nutmeg seed

Serves 4
per serving
Calories: 96
Protein: 6g
Carbs: 5g
Fat: 5g
Sat: 2g

    Bring zucchini and broth to boil in heavy medium saucepan. Reduce heat to medium-low, cover and simmer until zucchini is very tender, about 15 minutes.

    Working in batches, puree soup (or use an immersion blender...sort of a soup "outboard motor") on low in a blender until smooth. Return soup to same saucepan. Add cream, fresh nutmeg; stir over medium heat to prevent curdling. Season with sea salt and pepper.

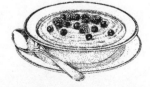

YELLOW TOMATO GAZPACHO

Serves 4
per serving
Calories: 217
Protein: 2g
Carbs: 12g
Fat: 20g
Sat: 2g

With so many heirloom tomatoes available today, here is an interesting take on an old favorite.

8 large yellow tomatoes
1/2 white onion
2 shallots
7 garlic cloves
1 tablespoon lemon juice
1 tablespoon sea salt
1/4 teaspoon black pepper
1 seeded yellow bell pepper
1/3 cup olive oil

Set olive oil aside. Mix all ingredients in large mixing bowl. Mix and puree in a blender in small batches. Add the olive oil slowly into the blender. Adjust seasonings and serve.

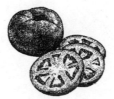

LEMON-DILL COD

Polluck, a relative of cod, is another good choice, as both fish are delicately flavored.

1/3 cup minced fresh dill
1/4 cup fresh lemon juice
1 tablespoon extra-virgin olive oil
4 teaspoons Dijon mustard
1/4 teaspoon sea salt
1/4 teaspoon freshly ground black pepper
4 (6-ounce) white fish fillets, such as pollock or cod

Serves 4
per serving
Calories: 166
Protein: 30g
Carbs: 0g
Fat: 5g
Sat: 1g

Combine all ingredients in a large zip-top plastic bag; seal and marinate in refrigerator 20 minutes. Remove fish from bag and discard marinade.

Place fish on a brill rack or broiler pan coated with cooking spray or misted olive oil. Cook for 4 minutes on each side or until fish flakes easily when tested with a fork.

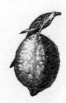

SPICY GRILLED CATFISH

Serves 4
per serving
Calories: 265
Protein: 22g
Carbs: 6g
Fat: 13g
Sat: 2g

2 teaspoons extra-virgin olive oil
1/4 cup lime juice
1 cup Chardonnay wine
2 tablespoons dry mustard
2 tablespoons chili powder
2 teaspoons pepper
1/2 cup chopped, fresh cilantro
1 pound catfish fillets

Preheat broiler.

Mix everything but the fillets in a bowl. Pour half of the marinade into another bowl and reserve for basting. Add catfish to the first bowl; marinate for 15 minutes.

Drain fillets and discard marinade from the first bowl. Place fillets on an oiled grill rack or broiler pan rack. Grill or broil 4 inches from the heat source, basting with reserved marinade, for about 3 minutes on each side, or until fish flakes easily with a fork.

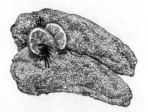

GRILLED SWORDFISH WITH SALSA VERDE

Grilling is a great way to cook meaty swordfish or halibut. Use 1/2-inch-thick steaks. You can also sear roast either fish for 7 minutes if you don't have access to a grill.

Serves 4
per serving
Calories: 248
Protein: 36g
Carbs: 3g
Fat: 10g
Sat: 2g

Salsa Verde
1/2 cup (tightly packed) fresh flat-leaf parlsey leaves
2 tablespoons drained capers
1 tablespoon Dijon mustard
1 large garlic clove
2 teaspoons extra-virgin olive oil
1 1/2 tablespoons fresh lemon juice
sea salt
1/2 teaspoon freshly ground pepper
Four 8-ounce swordfish steaks, cut 1/2 inch thick

Make the salsa verde by combining all the ingredients except the swordfish in a food processor or blender. Proccess until very finely minced, but not completely smooth.

If sear-roasting, heat the oven to 500 degrees and mist a metal baking pan with olive oil and place the swordfish steaks on the pan. Roast for 5 minutes. If using a grill, oil the grill and grill the steaks for 2 minutes per side, basting occasionally with olive oil, until just cooked through. Transfer to a large platter and serve with the salsa verde.

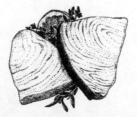

SKEWERED SHRIMP WITH FENNEL AND ORANGE

Serves 4
per serving
Calories: 188
Protein: 25g
Carbs: 17g
Fat: 4g
Sat: 1g

This is a Sicilian way to cook shrimp, which is luscious and fragrant. It works equally well with scallops. For a wonderful aroma, soak bay leaves in boiling water for about 30 minutes, until softened. Thread them between the oranges and peppers for a deep, almost haunting flavor. Here's another serving tip: Bake acorn squash, scoop out the seeds and use each half as a "boat" to serve your grilled shrimp.

2 teaspoons extra-virgin olive oil
2 tablespoons fennel seeds, ground
grated zest of 2 oranges
grated zest of 1 lemon
1/4 teaspoon crushed red pepper
1 pound large shrimp, shelled and deveined
2 medium fennel bulbs- halved, cored and cut into
    1-inch chunks, thick layers separated
2 medium red onions, cut into 1-inch chunks
3 medium oranges, halved lengthwise and
    sliced crosswise 1/3 inch thick
sea salt

In a small bowl, combine the olive oil, fennel seeds, grated orange and lemon zests and the crushed pepper.

Thread the shrimp, fennel, onions and oranges onto 4 metal skewers. Arrange the skewers in a shallow baking dish and brush them with the marinade. Cover and refrigerate for 3 to 4 hours, turning occasionally.

On a heated grill, cook the shrimp skewers for about 2 minutes per side, brushing occasionally with any remaining marinade, until the shrimp turn pink. Sprinkle lightly with salt and serve.

RED SNAPPER EN PAPILLOTE

Now that Reynold's Wrap has come out with foil cooking bags, this French technique is a "snap" to make. You can substitute leeks for fennel and add some tomatoes for a Mediterranean flavor.

Serves 4
per serving
Calories: 249
Protein: 38g
Carbs: 17g
Fat: 3g
Sat: 1g

4 tablespoons capers
4 tablespoons whole green peppercorns, drained
1 teaspoon dill seed
4 tablespoons freshly squeezed lemon juice
    (about 2 lemons)
2 fennel bulbs (about 1 1/2 pounds),
    thinly sliced lengthwise
Four 6-ounce red-snapper fillets, thinly sliced,
    boned and skinned
sea salt
1 lemon, cut into 8 thin slices

Heat oven to 400 degrees. Place two baking sheets in the oven. Combine the capers, peppercorns, dill seed, and lemon juice in a small bowl. Set aside.

Divide the fennel evenly between four Reynold's Wrap bags, forming a bed on one side. Sprinkle each serving with 1 tablespoon of the caper mixture; season with salt. Place a snapper fillet on each bed of fennel. Seal. Place packets on heated baking sheets. Back until puffed and fish is cooked, about 15 to 18 minutes. Transfer packets to individual plates and serve.

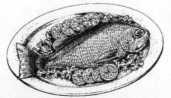

GRILLED HALIBUT STEAKS

Serves 4
per serving
Calories: 277
Protein: 47g
Carbs: 1g
Fat: 8g
Sat: 1g

1 clove garlic, minced
2 tablespoons sweet paprika
1 teaspoon ground cumin
1 teaspoon fresh lemon juice
1 tablespoon extra-virgin olive oil
sea salt, fresh pepper
Four 4- to 5-ounce halibut fillets, about 3/4 inch thick
lemon wedges for serving

In a small bowl, combine the garlic, paprika and cumin. Stir in the lemon juice, then add the olive oil and a pinch of sea salt and fresh black pepper. Arrange the fish in a 9-by-13-inch glass baking dish and rub the paste all over the fillets. Cover and refrigerate for at least 4 up to 8 hours.

Light the grill or preheat the broiler. Transfer fillets to a pan. Season the fish with another pinch of sea salt and pepper. Grill or broil the halibut for about 3 minutes per side, until just cooked through. Transfer to a platter and serve garnished with lemon wedges.

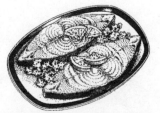

THAI WATERFALL SALAD

This is a wonderful dish that blends the juices from the meat with wonderful flavors that create a "waterfall" when mixed, dressing the vegetables. You can use grilled beef or pork for a different variation.

Serves 4
per serving
Calories: 171
Protein: 17g
Carbs: 16g
Fat: 5g
Sat: 1g

3/4 pound beef skirt steak (or ground pork
    or lean ground beef)
sea salt
freshly ground black pepper
1 cup Thai basil leaves, (also known as "holy" basil),
    torn into pieces
1/4 cup mint leaves, torn into pieces
1 red onion, thinly sliced
1 cucumber, peeled, seeded and thinly sliced
1/2 cup cilantro leaves, coarsely chopped
1/2 cup lime juice
1/4 cup fish sauce, or to taste
1 tablespoon dried red pepper flakes
pinch sugar

Season steak with salt and pepper and grill over medium-high heat until browned, 30 seconds each side. Let rest 5 minutes before slicing against the grain into 1/4 inch slices. (If using ground meat, saute on low heat to extract more juices. Place meat and juices in a bowl.)

Combine warm meat with the remaining ingredients, working them between your fingers to blend.

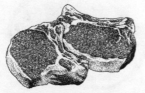

BAY WATCH TURKEY BURGERS

Serves 2
per serving
Calories: 334
Protein: 38g
Carbs: 5g
Fat: 18g
Sat: 7g

Want to discover how those sand studs on "Bay Watch" keep such a great physique? It's in the meat. We all know how dry ground turkey can be, but placing a tablespoon of Boursin cheese (especially the peppered version) between the patty makes this meal glisten with taste!

1/2 small red onion
3/4 pound ground turkey
2 tablespoons Boursin cheese

Prepare grill.

Finely chop onion. In a bowl, gently combine onion and turkey (do not over-mix) and form into four 1/2-inch-thick patties. Center 1 tablespoon Boursin on each of 2 patties and top with remaining 2 patties, pressing edges together to seal. Season burgers with sea salt and pepper and grill on a lightly oiled rack until just cooked through.

ASPARAGUS THE BARBARIAN

Serves 4
per serving
Calories: 16
Protein: 3g
Carbs: 1g
Fat: 1g
Sat: 0g

When this vegetable is in season, there is nothing better than strong, thick stalks of asparagus given a quick broiling. It's guaranteed to bring out the barbarian in your man.

1 pound thick asparagus spears, cleaned and trimmed
Mister with extra-virgin olive oil
sea salt

Preheat oven to 500 degrees.

Trim asparagus spears. Mist a baking sheet with olive oil and layer asparagus single file. Do not crowd them. Mist the spears with olive oil and grind sea salt over them. Place in the oven on the middle rack and roast for 7 minutes. Remove from the pan and allow to come to room temperature before serving.

LEMON CHICKEN KABOBS

These are equally good cold or hot, so make extra.

1 pound chicken breast, cut into chunks
1/3 cup peanut oil
1 teaspoon lemon juice
1 teaspoon red wine vinegar
2 tablespoons seasoning mix (composed of equal
    amounts whole marjoram, thyme, oregano, basil
    leaves, ground pepper)
sea salt
1 clove garlic, minced
lemon wedges

*Serves 4
per serving
(2 skewers):*
Calories: 291
Protein: 17g
Carbs: 0g
Fat: 16g
Sat: 3g

In a blender container place oil, lemon juice, vinegar, spice mixture and garlic. Blend on high for 30 seconds.

Place chicken chunks in a large plastic bag and pour marinade over chicken and marinate in the refrigerator overnight. Remove chicken from marinade and drain well.

Thread on skewers, alternating 3 chunks of chicken and 2 lemon wedges per skewer. Grill about 4 minutes per side. Serve immediately or chill in refrigerator and serve cold.

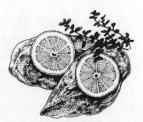

DRUNKEN CHICKEN ON A CAN

Serves 4
per serving
Calories: 215
Protein: 32g
Carbs: 0g
Fat: 8g
Sat: 3g

This is such a ridiculously easy way to prepare chicken, I had to include it. You can make it either on the BBQ or in the oven...just choose a chicken about 4 pounds in size if you want the can to fit.

One 4 pound chicken
3 tablespoon spice rub (choose any brand – Emeril's,
      Lawry's or your favorite blend)
One 12 ounce can of beer

Heat the oven to 350 degrees.

Have your frat boy drink about 1/4 cup of the beer. With churchkey can opener, punch two other holes in the top.

Season chicken under the skin with the spice rub. Slide chicken over the can so that the drumsticks reach down to bottom of can and chicken stands upright (like a vertical roaster).

Place the chicken in a pie plate upright and roast for 1 hour.

Transfer chicken when done to a platter and THROW AWAY THE BEER!

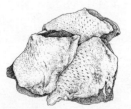

CHAPTER 5
Testosterone: Forever Strong, Forever Young

It's the Holy Grail of manhood...the stuff that causes men to go to war, plot corporate takeovers, watch Wrestlemania, race cars too fast and act like they truly ARE from Mars! It's the new estrogen for men in the gray zone, the illusive fountain of youth. It's testosterone. The word evokes images of chiseled gladiators, gleaming with sweat in a Roman arena. Pound for pound, testosterone can cause more aggressiveness, energy, confidence and lust than a sighting of Pamela Anderson at the beach. Though testosterone was first isolated in 1935, research has been slow. Hormone-replacement therapy is one of the few areas of medicine where research on men lags behind that on women.

Testosterone is an androgen, or male hormone that is produced both in the adrenals and testes of men. Though women produce this same steroid from their ovaries and adrenals, the average male pumps out 260-1000 nanograms of testosterone per deciliter of blood plasma, dwarfing the minuscule 15-70 nanograms a woman gets to play around with in her body. But not all this testosterone is pure hormonal gold. Just how much is free to circulate and cause that morning Johnson is an individual matter.

Testosterone is what, in utero, turns a few dividing cells into boys. During the first few weeks after conception, all embryos are capable of being either female or male. Around the sixth week, the Y chromosome (found only in males) triggers a surge of testosterone, which sets in motion the formation of a penis and testes along with the ability to play bongo drums on your bladder. During adolescence, another eruption of testosterone occurs, turning sweet, angelic boys into hairy hulks with blood testosterone levels as high as 2000 nanograms. This hormonal kegger triggers increased levels of aggressiveness, muscle growth and a need to steal girl's panties. So what's not to love?

Animal studies have repeatedly shown that testosterone, competition and aggression go hand in hand. Castrate an animal and you get a pussycat, but give the same creature just 20% of his testosterone back and he resumes his wild cat behavior. Give him too much and he'll send your bunny slippers running for cover! It's all about domination and competition for a mate. In the primal world, where procreation is king, even feral fowl will eject the sperm of subdominant, lower testosterone males in favor of the alpha or dominant ones.[144] Sex may make the world go 'round but it's testosterone that's turning the crankshaft.

Testosterone (T) levels fluctuate in healthy men, peaking around 8 a.m. and dropping almost in half by evening. Coincidentally, this is exactly the pattern of cortisol production. Overall T levels remain fairly constant until age 30, when levels can drop as much as 1 percent a year in some men. Middle-age men who preserve the body weight they had in their 20's may not experience any fall-off in production, while overweight adult males of any age tend to have lower testosterone levels.

Overweight adult males of any age tend to have lower testosterone levels

MALE MENOPAUSE

Damage to either the Leydig cells in the testicles or to the hypothalamus can put a damper on T production. Infections, alcohol, lifestyle, trauma or AIDS are just a few of the roadblocks on the hypothalamic-pituitary-gonadal highway. And when

T levels drop, so does a man's sex drive and his ability not only to achieve, but to maintain an erection. Unlike women, who experience lowered estrogen levels in response to fewer eggs left in their ovaries, men at any age can suddenly find themselves converting valuable testosterone into estrogen. How does that happen? Through an enzyme system contained in fat cells and in the liver called aromatase.

Like testosterone in the female, the window of optimum effectiveness for estrogen in men is very small. It doesn't take much to cause estrogen to switch off the activities of testosterone. In older men, however, this elevation can semi-permanently accelerate aging as aromatase levels increase and a man's ability to excrete or inactivate estrogen decline. As a result, men become over-estrogenized, throwing the ratio of testosterone to estrogen so out of balance you've got Sherman Klump instead of Don Juan!

GOING TO SEED

Producing too much estrogen can cause infertility in young men. When 106 men under the age of 40 were evaluated as partners of an infertile couple, 65% had elevated cholesterol and triglyceride levels and nearly half were overweight by clinical standards. Not surprisingly, they also were glucose intolerant, hypertensive and found to have estradiol levels exceeding 50 pg/ml.[145] There's little doubt these men won't be around to bounce grandchildren on their knees if they remain this unhealthy!

IS HE GOING SOFT?

A young swashbuckler may have a ratio of 50/1 when it comes to testosterone/estrogen balance, but by the time he is a one-eyed old pirate, this value could have changed to 20/1 or possibly lower. Even though testosterone production may slow with aging, the rise in estrogen is far more significant to his health. Estrogen can increase his risk for a heart attack, diabetes, stroke and impotency.[146] It can enlarge his prostate, making urination so slow he can't write his name in the snow. How does it get this way? Let me show you the seven enemies of your's man's potency and health.

MOST UNWANTED LIST

1) Obesity

That's right. Just being overweight by as little as ten pounds, will increase the estrogen in their systems. The more fat cells they have, the more little aromatase factories are happily converting testosterone into estrogen with no regard for age. The most active units are the fat cells hidden deep inside the abdomen, the ones that can snuggle up against the liver, releasing fatty acids into the blood stream while picking up additional fat for storage. This results in an elevation of the bad cholesterol that can clog small blood vessels, especially the ones in the penis responsible for maintaining erection. Remember, having a waistline of 42 inches instead of 32 inches significantly tilts the testosterone/estrogen balance in the wrong direction, doubling the risk for impotency in men of any age.[3]

2) Liver function

The liver processes and directs elimination of hormones and drugs from the body. As we age, the enzymatic function of our livers slows, leading to weight gain and lowers the efficiency with which we handle the byproducts of our hormones. In men, this results in a gradual buildup of estrogen. Metabolism changes can occur because of alcohol and drugs. In fact, a slowing in the CP450 pathway, the main fuel box of the liver, is considered one of the most important signs of aging.

3) Aromatase activity

As the CP450 enzyme pathway ages, it produces more aromatase, the enzyme responsible for converting testosterone into estrogen. Now add obesity, and you've got an entire sweat shop manufacturing estrogen with the help of this enzyme.

4) Zinc deficiency

It's hard to believe that a little mineral, such as zinc, could be so critical to a man's potency. Zinc can nuke a man's aromatase production, resulting in higher testosterone levels. In return, it takes a normal amount of testosterone to maintain levels of zinc within tissues such as the Leydig cells in the testicles.[147] Without zinc, the pituitary is unable to send signals to the testicles to produce more testosterone. Even short term losses in zinc can reduce a guy's semen volume, sperm count and testosterone, making conception difficult.[148,149] I'm sure it wouldn't surprise you to learn the average American diet is low in zinc, especially among the elderly. Again, alcohol and medications, such as diuretics, can be responsible for this outcome.[150]

5) Alcohol

Alcohol slows down and even damages the CP450 enzyme system in the liver and can lower zinc levels. Add it's ability to raise estrogen production and you've got a hormonal hat trick. Even Shakespeare realized that "alcohol provokes the desire but takes away the performance." Alcohol has a direct toxic effect on the testicles and can lower testosterone concentrations in men even if they don't drink chronically. [151,152]

6) Drugs

Medication and recreational drugs can lower testosterone and raise the ratio of estrogen produced in a man's body.[153] Chronic marijuana use can even enlarge a man's breasts. Medication, such as diuretics, antibiotics and antihypertensives, can diminish testosterone production by either affecting the CP450 enzymes or lowering blood zinc levels. Smoking cigarettes not only torches sexual desire and performance but can also increase estrogen levels in men. And if he inhales marijuana, he can quadruple his chances of dropping dead from a heart attack within the first hour after lighting up.[154-156] No wonder James Bond kicked the habit as he matured!

7) Licorice and Stevia

That's right...the sticky kind that turns your teeth black at Halloween. This food product raises blood pressure higher than Ali McBeal's skirts by blocking the conversion of cortisol to cortisone, the less active form. While researchers once thought it took mass quantities of licorice to cause this effect, recent studies show as little as 50 gm a day (about the size of a few jellybeans) can increase your blood pressure as much as 5 points.[157] But in an even more startling effect, just 7 gm of licorice (less than an ounce, the amount found in a few cough drops or breath mints) can slice testosterone levels. Black licorice contains glycyrrhizic acid, which prevents conversion of progesterone to androstenedione. This sweet stuff can sour a man's libido, resulting in more than a 34% drop in testosterone levels.[158] Licorice is used in tobacco (cigarettes and chewing tobacco) and dark beers, so avoiding it can be a sticky situation. And speaking of sweet things...stevia is another herb that works better than salt peter at dropping testosterone levels.[159] This natural sweetener blocks an androgen receptor in the testicles. When rats were fed stevia, their testicles actually shrank in size. So if you want your man to have good n' plenty testosterone, avoid these products.

HE'S ALL BOUND UP

With all this talk about estrogen, aromatase and the CP450 system, we are really talking about how many ways a man can sabotage his own testosterone. But there's more to this story, as not all testosterone is available to work it's hormonal magic. A lot of testosterone is bound to a protein in the blood called sex hormone binding globulin, or SHBG. Levels of this protein increase with age and coincidentally are stimulated by estrogen. High levels of testosterone actually inhibit SHBG production and allow more testosterone to "go free"...about 2 to 3 percent...and that's platinum to a man's sexual function. So a middle-aged man who wants to remain a gladiator might face several opponents in his battle to maintain virility, health and strength. To sustain a normal weight he needs testosterone, but in reality, his testosterone levels are starting to drop, which causes him to gain weight. Fat increases the amount of estrogen he manufactures from his testosterone and that stimulates more SHBG, which cages his free testosterone, which leads to MORE estrogen production. Now add alcohol, smoking and medications that affect his metabolism or lower his zinc levels, and those aromatase fat factories start spinning hormonal gold into fraying straw.

HOLY MACHO MAN!

So how can a man keep that critical edge? Scientists are hotly debating the issue, but the consensus seems to be heading in the direction of hormone replacement therapy for men. That's right ...men may actually experience a male menopause unique to their own personal metabolism. In other words, it's not necessarily related to a specific age range, but rather a set of conditions which band together to lower the amount of available free testosterone while increasing the percentage of circulating estrone and estradiol.

This means a man could experience "premature menopause" just like a woman if he sports a physique with loads of fat squatting on his frame. This would increase his risk for cardiac disease, high blood pressure, diabetes, strokes and impotency. Conversely, by keeping his weight under control he may produce enough free testosterone to protect his heart and both his heads.

Hypothyroid men complain of decreased sex drive

MOST ELIGIBLE MEN

So who should be evaluated for testosterone replacement therapy (TRT)? Men who suffer from the following medical conditions may be prime candidates for therapy.

1) Thyroid disease

Thyroxin can affect a man's virility by altering the amount of free testosterone available to his tissues. Over 14% of men have mild thyroid failure or subclinical hypothyroidism. In addition, men with this condition have elevated cholesterol levels in direct proportion to the elevation in their thyroid stimulating hormone.[160] When a man is hypothyroid, leutenizing hormone and follicle stimulating hormone are high. This makes the testicles resist signals from the pituitary. Serum testosterone and SHBG usually decrease, while free testosterone may be low, normal or high. Over 60% of men who are hypothyroid complain of decreased sex drive.[161] Just giving him thyroxin, however, will not stimulate his sex drive, correct any erectile problems nor necessarily lower his cholesterol. Low free testosterone may be a contributing factor to some of the signs and symptoms of hypothyroidism.[162] To learn more about this condition, I suggest you read "Living Well with

Hypothyroidism: What Your Doctor Doesn't Tell You...That You Need to Know" by Mary Shomon.

2) Metabolic Syndrome

Researchers have identified a cluster of symptoms which put a man at high risk for developing heart disease. Known as Metabolic Syndrome X, it is characterized by men with two or more of the following conditions: insulin resistance with resulting elevated insulin levels, elevated lipids (especially triglycerides), high uric acid levels, obesity and hypertension. Not surprisingly, it is associated with low testosterone.[10,11,163] Men with this condition may benefit from T replacement therapy, as coronary artery disease has been shown to be the result of low, not high levels of T.[7] When men with angina (chest pain brought on by cardiovascular disease) were given T replacement therapy, blood flow to their hearts improved.[164]

Looking for a sign your man may be at risk for heart disease? Just take a peek at the back of his head. Men who have the tonsured look of a monk have a 36% greater risk of heart disease than a guy with frontal or temporal balding.[6] What's hair today could be gone tomorrow!

3) Diabetes

Men with diabetes have less free testosterone to help maintain their blood sugar and insulin balance.[165] This leads to increased risk for heart disease, strokes and impotency. Not surprisingly, more than 50% of diabetic men have problems with erections by the time they reach age 60.[166] Difficulty with morning and spontaneous erections was the most common complaint.[167]

4) Erectile dysfunction (ED)

Impotency has many causes, and not all are due to changes in testosterone production. However, ED, especially when it has a vascular basis, can be a "yellow flag" warning men they may be silently experiencing heart disease as well. Researchers in the Massachusetts Male Aging Study evaluated 57 men with ED who had no signs or risk factors for hypertension, diabetes, arterial disease or high cholesterol. Sixty percent were found to have elevated cholesterol and 91% had abnormal blood flow to the penis.[168] Now your gladiator has turned into a gladiola because the blood vessels that supply the penis are narrower than arteries in other parts of the body. Cholesterol plaques may cause obstruction in the penis before they obstruct slightly larger arteries, such as those in the heart.[169,170]

FIRST CLASS MALE

Nocturnal erections are the earliest ones to change, but unless you stay up all night with a flashlight, you won't know if he's having a hard time or not. Here's a proven method that has been studied repeatedly and found to be first class: simply apply a ring of postage stamps around the base of the penis at bedtime. If the stamp ring is unbroken by morning, your man is suffering from erectile dysfunction.[171-173] This test is highly accurate, not to mention sensitive.[174] The only argument may be who gets to lick the stamps.

5) Obesity

Packing on the pounds, especially if a man is more than 25 pounds overweight, can mean a boatload of trouble. Stuffing his abdomen with fat creates a belly full of toxic weight that can be an indication of low testosterone or an out-of-whack T/estradiol ratio.[175,176] The combination of obesity AND low testosterone puts men at greatest risk for heart disease.[31] As discussed earlier, it is part of the Metabolic Syndrome X profile. In a recent study, obesity was up a whopping 54 percent among young adults between the ages of 30-39, leading to a 70% increase in Type 2 diabetes.[177] Not only does diabetes cause heart disease and impotency, but it is the leading cause of blindness.

6) Age

As long ago as 1944, researchers recognized that testosterone deficiency can cause depression, insomnia, headaches, muscle pains and fatigue, not to mention sending a man's sex drive into a nose dive. Just surviving life can result in one's liver producing more testosterone-converting aromatase enzymes, which in turn bumps up a man's estrogen levels. So if your warrior is experiencing mid-life health problems, he needs to investigate his testosterone levels.

7) Osteoporosis

Approximately 2 million men in the United States have osteoporosis or brittle bones, and another 13 million have bones which contain less than the desirable amount of calcium.[178,179] This puts men at risk for vertebral and hip fractures, especially if they can't or don't exercise.[180] Low free testosterone whittles away at a man's muscle mass, making him twice as likely to die from a hip fracture as is a woman.[181-183]

8) Depression

Feeling moody and down in the dumps may be more than a mid-life crisis. Men who suffer from depression may have low free testosterone levels, making them irritable, nervous, angry and sad.[184,185] When free T levels were restored to normal, so were their feelings of energy, friendliness and well-being.[186]

Now that you know the indications for TRT, does it matter in which form it is given?

FORMAT MATTERS

The format in which testosterone supplementation is delivered has a critical impact on a man's health, as no other hormone in his body can be replaced by as many other types of hormones than testosterone. Like ERT for women, TRT comes in all shapes and sizes...shots, creams, pills, patches, pellets and gels, but very few have the format to prevent rapid metabolism into estradiol.

Give a man a "shot" of the Big T and his testosterone levels rise quickly but fail to mimic the natural circadian rhythm that results in higher levels of T in the morning versus night. His levels may be too high initially, up to 1400ng/dl, making him feel hostile, aggressive, even combative. This roller coaster quickly drops as testosterone is converted to estrogen. Remember...nature intended estrogen to act as the brake on too much testosterone in men. Now he's lost that "loving feeling" and feels depressed, fatigued and out of sorts. No wonder women view men on this kind of therapy with the same affection china shopkeepers have for a bull.

When it comes to pills, convenience is really their only asset. Oral T is absorbed rapidly from the GI tract and circulates through the liver. This allows only a small amount of T to circulate without raising estradiol or another hormone, DHT. However, there is significant liver damage from the type of testosterone available in the United States. Again, Europe is ahead of us and has approved an oral preparation, testosterone undecanoate, which is partially absorbed by the lymph system, bypassing the liver. This compound, when given in divided doses of 120 to 240 mg/d brings T levels back to normal without raising estrogen above normal ranges.

Patches avoid unusually high levels of T and help to restore the normal diurnal T pattern. But here is where things get hairy. One patch is made for the scrotum, requiring shaving and an unusual manner of straightening out the wrinkles in order for the appliance to stick. I don't even want to mention removal, which can only be described as invented by the Marquis de Sade. This patch is applied in the evening, resulting in normal morning values that taper off by nighttime.

The slower testosterone is presented to the body, the less estrogen is produced

Fortunately, another patch has been approved, called Androderm, which can be applied anywhere BUT the scrotum and also maintains a diurnal blood concentration of testosterone, estradiol and DHT. Like estrogen patches for women, some men may be allergic to the adhesive and develop "hickies" wherever one is applied.

Pellets are widely used in Europe, but again, are not generally available in the US. The pellets need only be implanted every 3-4 months and are embedded in body fat much the same way pellet therapy for women is done. The testosterone gradually dissolves, which prevents unusually high levels of T from turning on the estrogen pathway. The slower T is presented to the body, the less estrogen is produced. Bartor Pharmacal in Rye, New York manufactures testosterone pellets.

Creams and gels are an excellent way to adjust T levels, as they can be applied in a diurnal pattern and are easily absorbed without the above mentioned "tatoo". AndroGel, the new "swell" gell, is slowly absorbed, resulting in lower conversion rates of testosterone to estrogen. However, it can cause hair growth and even raise testosterone levels in women coming in contact with a man's coated skin. The answer? Advise him to take a shower 30 minutes after application. Gels and creams are easy to overdose, especially if your man is the type that prefers to rub them all over his body like sun tan lotion during Spring break. So remind him this is one format where too much is NOT a good thing.

GETTING IT RIGHT

By now you've realized that adjusting testosterone levels is an imperfect science, but there is a zone that appears to be right for most men. When researchers studied over 4,000 men between ages 32 to 44, the healthiest men had total testosterone levels between 400 and 600 nannograms. These men had less chance of having high blood pressure or heart disease and were 75 percent less likely to be obese.[187] Those with T levels over 1,000 were prone to engage in risky behavior and unlikely to reap the positive benefits of testosterone. Drop a man below 400 and he complains of aches and pains in his joints, ED, poor strength, vanishing stamina and a lack of mental aggressiveness.

Table 8 summarizes the desirable ranges of total T, free T and estradiol for a healthy man. Remember, he doesn't want to marinate in testosterone, just baste with the right amount in order to remain strong and virile. Like ERT levels for women, testosterone levels need to be monitored, as acne, breast enlargement, or an elevated blood hematocrit could be signs of too much testosterone.

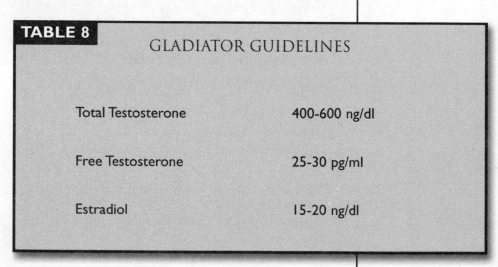

TABLE 8	GLADIATOR GUIDELINES
Total Testosterone	400-600 ng/dl
Free Testosterone	25-30 pg/ml
Estradiol	15-20 ng/dl

THE GOOD, THE BAD AND THE UGLY

Although testosterone replacement therapy can put the swagger back into a hormone-deficient man's step, it shouldn't be used to reverse the signs of aging in a men with normal testosterone levels. Like all things, TRT has a good, bad and ugly side to it, resulting in the following changes:

1) Suppression of sperm count

Testosterone is important to the production of sperm, but when given as a hormone, it actually suppresses the production of semen after about 10 weeks. In fact, researchers are looking into T therapy as a form of male birth control pill. The good news is that sperm levels and fertility return to normal within six to 18 months after stopping T therapy.[188]

2) Lipid changes

Keeping testosterone levels within the normal range is known to reduce cholesterol and the bad lipoproteins, or LDL, but some men can drop the good cholesterol (HDL) and raise their blood viscosity, which can lead to strokes and heart disease. If your warrior is taking TRT, he should have his lipid values followed as part of his regular check-up.[189]

3) Sleep apnea

A man may absorb too little oxygen at night because of sleep apnea, causing an unhealthy rise in his blood hematocrit. This condition of snoring with episodes of breath holding, is found when testosterone and estradiol levels are elevated.[190] Remember, the format in which testosterone is delivered is all-important to how rapidly testosterone is converted to estrogen in a man's body. Studies showed the patch or gel resulted in the fewest cases of this type of change.[191]

4) Prostate changes and cancer

It may surprise you to know that a PSA test is

NOT specific for cancer of the prostate, but rather is a good test for judging the effects of male hormones on the prostate. When men were given testosterone therapy, their prostates actually shrank in comparison to men low in testosterone.[192] There's also little proof that TRT causes prostate cancer. In fact, recent studies show no apparent relationship between T and the incidence of prostate cancer.[193,194] However, if a man already has cancer of the prostate, testosterone can spread the disease. It's wise to request a PSA test and prostate ultrasound before beginning any form of hormone therapy.

The information I have given you in this chapter is cutting edge, so don't be discouraged if your gladiator's doctor hasn't read all of these studies or isn't familiar with the differences in formats. Just understand that TRT can benefit men with low testosterone due to a myriad of conditions. After all, who wouldn't want to feel all spit, chromed and polished in life. So let's take a look at the non-hormonal ways he can build a nutritional armory to protect his health.

CHAPTER 6
The Gladiator's Nutritional Armory

By now you should be certain of two things: First, a gladiator wants a muscular, lean and fit body. Second, he shouldn't sacrifice his health to achieve it. Follow The Gladiator Diet, and you improve your warrior's vitamin balance by feeding him nutritionally dense foods. However, since you will be eliminating many of the processed "fortified" grains and starches, you'll need to make sure you replace these nutrients if you want to keep his testosterone within a normal and reasonable range.

- **Zinc (as zinc picolinate) —50mg**

    In recent years, zinc has finally been recognized as a very important nutrient in growth and healing. The bitter metallic taste in your mouth when you eat iodinated table salt is caused by the interaction of zinc in your saliva with the iodine. This metal is important to carbohydrate, fat and protein metabolism and can help your man's immune system fight off a cold. It can even help him switch off that craving for starchy, high sugar carbohydrates.[195]

    Zinc is crucial for testosterone production and metabolism. Blood and testicular testosterone in young men fed a diet low in zinc fell through the floor in just five weeks.[148] Too much calcium can do the same thing. Diets high in calcium or calcium-containing supplements can block absorption of zinc from the gut, so go easy on dairy products. When serum zinc levels rise, plasma testosterone and muscular development increase.[147,149,196] Insulin-like growth factor (IGF-I) is a critical element in bone formation and protein metabolism, and is lowered by zinc deficiency, which contributes to osteoporosis. Thiazide diuretics and alcohol can aggravate zinc deficiency and increase the amount of testosterone converted to estrogen. This contributes to impotency. The mighty oyster is a veritable zinc grenade, but other foods high in this mineral include meat and poultry (especially dark meat), shellfish and legumes.

- Folic acid—500mg

    One of the B vitamins, folic acid lowers blood levels of homocysteine, a risk factor for atherosclerotic disease. A simple deficiency in this vitamin may trigger 30 to 40% of the heart attacks and strokes suffered in America.[197] In a study of folate intake and its effect on homocysteine levels, researchers found the current RDA of 180 micrograms/day failed to keeps levels of this amino acid low, and they recommended an intake of 516 micrograms/day to decrease the levels of homocysteine.[198] Folic acid can also protect against cancer by altering DNA changes in white blood cells. Good sources for folate are liver, nuts, lentils, spinach and other dark leafy greens, oranges and avocados. For the best availability of folate, choose fresh produce from a farmer's market or the organic section of your grocery store.

- Vitamin E —400 iu

    D-alpha tocopherol is a powerful antioxidant which acts like a bug zapper to protect the first line of defense of any cell – its membrane. Vitamin E, which is fat soluble, helps keep the good cholesterol (HDL) high while lowering the bad cholesterol (LDL), and can reduce swelling from arthritis while slowing the development of cataracts. Good sources are peanut butter, liver, leafy greens, soybeans and nuts. Daily dosages above 800iu may cause hypertension. Since freezing destroys the activity of vitamin E in vegetables, it's best to eat them fresh.

- Vitamin C—1000mg

    It has been touted as the miracle vitamin, a cure for everything from the common cold to cancer. Ascorbic acid (Vitamin C) can reduce the risk of gallbladder disease and stones by altering the breakdown of cholesterol.[199-201] Moderate Vitamin C levels are associated with a reduction in heart disease and stroke.[202] Vitamin C is a vital piece in a gladiator's nutritional armory because it enhances the pituitary gland's response to changes in testosterone levels.[203] Conversely, low levels can boost levels of aromatase, the principle agent for converting testosterone to estrogen.[204] Good sources are fresh fruits, melons, strawberries, broccoli, sweet red and green peppers, tomatoes, brussels sprouts, cabbage and dark leafy greens like chard, kale, collards, spinach, mustard and turnips. The darker and brighter the green pigment, the more Vitamin C inside.

- Pyridoxal-5-phosphate—20mg

    Pyridoxine, or B6, is essential for protein metabolism because it helps convert glycogen into glucose, which energizes your muscles. It is an important co-factor in the regulation of 26 aminotransferases, enzymes that regulate the proper pathways for our neuroendocrine system. B6 has the ability to decrease secretion of prolactin, an inhibitor of testosterone production. If your man is deficient in B6, he may form kidney stones when he eats sugars such as fructose or galactose.[205] B6 depletion disturbs the metabolism of tryptophan. This can cause depression, anxiety, decreased sex drive and impaired glucose tolerance.[206] B6 is important in lowering homocysteine levels in blood. Pyridoxal-5-phosphate, the liver metabolized form of B6, is the active component. However, men who are prone to herpetic outbreaks should not take B6 as it increases viral activity.

- **Arginine-1500 mg with ornithine**

   This amino acid can handcuff cholesterol and lower blood pressure. Arginine is found in the gelatinous material extracted from bone marrow. It's what gives chicken soup its medicinal properties. The jelly that congeals on a plate contains a growth factor which can slow the replication of viruses. More important, arginine and vitamin E can block the atherosclerotic plaques that cause blood vessels to spasm and deprive tissue of oxygen.[207] Arginine, especially L-arginine, restores the protective effects of cholecystokinin on the stomach lining.[208] It can also prevent damage to the kidneys by increasing the excretion of nitric oxide metabolites, which can scar the filtration units called glomeruli.[209] Arginine helps wounds heal from surgery by stimulating the immune system in surgical patients.[210] L-arginine stimulates growth hormone production and inhibits the effect of cortisol on his hormones.[211] A diet rich in carbohydrates has very little arginine, while a protein rich diet has oodles of this amino acid. Arginine can make one acidotic, so take it in combination with ornithine, another amino acid. Turkey, soybeans and chicken are pure meat zirconium and loaded with this amino acid. In fact, soy is exceptionally rich in arginine, compared to animal sources.

- **Alpha lipoic acid — 100mg**

   Alpha lipoic acid (ALA) is a great antioxidant that occurs naturally in our bodies and recycles

Vitamins C, E and glutathione. The accumulation of high levels of free radicals results in depletion of glutathione and destruction of cell membranes. This causes nucleic acid, or DNA changes. ALA interferes with biochemical and physical damage caused by free radicals recycling and generating additional glutathione. It also helps prevent atherosclerotic plaques from adhering to the lining of arteries. ALA is a co-enzyme to numerous processes that occur within the mitochondria, or energy powerhouse in each cell. It can attract copper like the tractor beam pull of the Enterprise, preventing this mineral from damaging cell walls, and can improve glucose transport into cells by altering insulin resistance.[212-214] Research continues into the many ways this coenzyme can help prevent aging, nerve damage and heart disease.

- Resveratrol—100mg
- Quercitin—1000mg

These recently-discovered extracts from grape skins are believed to be the key substances in wine that protect against heart disease. More importantly, these food concentrates stimulate the function of the CP450 enzyme system in the liver to remove excess estrogen from a man's body. Resveratrol, extracted from the grape seed, is nearly fifty times more potent than Vitamin E as an antioxidant. Only your mother-in-law has the same effect in such a small dose![215] It can even inhibit benign prostatic tissue growth.[216] Quercitin, another flavonoid, was found to improve irritative bladder symptoms in men with chronic abacterial prostatitis when combined with bromelain and papain, two enzymes found in papaya and pineapple.[217] High levels of metabolic byproducts of quercitin have been found in plasma, which accounts for its ability to prevent oxidative damage in the blood.[218]

- Soy—190mg isoflavones/week, 25gm soy protein/day

     Some phytoestrogens, like beans and soy, are high in protein. Just adding 25 gm of soy protein a day can lower cholesterol.[105] Forty milligrams of isoflavones per day, the equivalent of one serving of a soy food, equals the typical Asian diet.[219] That's about 2 tablespoons of soy powder or 1/4 of a vacuum-packed tofu container. Soy also helps block fat cells from converting androstene-dione into estrogen.[107] As an additional benefit, it can also inhibit tyrosine kinase, an enzyme that helps prostate cancer cells to multiply.[108] But don't serve massive amounts of soy, because isoflavones inhibit thyroid peroxidase, which makes T3 and T4. This can lead to thyroid abnormalities, including goiter, autoimmune thyroiditis and brain damage.[220-222] Recent studies recommend that men consume no more than 190mg of isoflavones a week. Unfortunately, products are not required to list the amount of soy protein or isoflavones in a serving. It is best to avoid supplements, which contain isolates in much higher quantities than found in normal soy products, such as tofu or tempeh.

- Saw Palmetto Extract — 120mg

     Serenoa repens, or saw palmetto berries, is an extract from a tropical palm-like plant. It has been touted as an aphrodisiac, as it is able to block the conversion of testosterone to DHT at certain target tissues.[223] It has anti-estrogenic properties and is helpful in preventing prostate tissue growth, much like Proscar.[224-226] Although it is available as a tea, water does not extract the fatty acids responsible for its beneficial effect.

The following vitamins and minerals are found in any good, general vitamin supplement and should be part of your warrior's nutritional armory:

- Selenium—200mcg

  This trace mineral functions in concert with Vitamin E to scavenge free radicals and heavy metals. It is thought to help in the prevention of cancer. It's also important for thyroid function, as it aids in converting T4 to T3. Good sources include Brazil nuts, eggs, lean meats, seafood and legumes.

- Magnesium—250mg

  This mineral acts to balance the solubility of calcium in urine and tissues. It is vital to metabolism and activates more than 300 different enzymes in the body, particularly those that need the B vitamins for action. It helps to prevent tooth decay by binding calcium to teeth. Good sources are avocados, green vegetables, chocolate (70% cocoa), legumes, nuts and seeds.

- Beta carotene—5000iu

  A precursor of Vitamin A, it is believed to reduce the risk of certain types of cancer. It's water soluble, which means if you give him too much he'll wind up nourishing your toilet bowl. Food sources such as dark orange fruits and vegetables, like winter squash, pack an amazing amount of beta carotene into a single serving.

- Vitamin D

  Cholecalciferol (Vitamin D) is God's gift from sunshine. It regulates phosphorus and calcium metabolism which is important for strong bones. Good sources are cod liver oil, dairy products, butter, eggs, liver, fish such as salmon and of course, sunshine.

- Biotin

  This is a high sulfur B vitamin which plays a key role in carbohydrate, fat and protein metabolism. It's what gives rotten eggs their odor! Biotin is important for healthy nails, hair and skin. Good sources are egg yolks, meats, liver, milk, nuts, legumes, peanut butter, chocolate and cauliflower.

- **Pantothenic acid**

    Its Greek name, means "do anything" and that's just about how it works. It's a key component to Coenzyme A, which is important to his metabolism of carbohydrates, fats and proteins. Good sources are most fish, but all food groups contain some pantothenic acid.

- **Riboflavin**

    It's nature's way of giving him the benefits of niacin without the "hot flashes." It's an important B vitamin in the metabolism of tryptophan and has been found to help prevent migraines.[227] Riboflavin is water-soluble and works with B6, folate and niacin to maintain the integrity of red blood cells. It also helps to metabolize carbohydrates, fats and proteins. Good sources are liver, eggs, milk, yogurt, cheese, dark green vegetables, spinach and broccoli.

- **Potassium**

    An important mineral in maintaining fluid balance. It also helps his body break down carbohydrates and protein. Good sources include fruits, vegetables, dairy products, fish, lean meats and poultry.

- **Chromium**

    Helps regulate cholesterol and fatty acid production by making the body more sensitive to insulin. It also aids in the digestion of protein. Good sources are unpeeled apples, oysters, nuts, peanut butter, liver and meat.

- **Manganese**

   A trace element that appears in a variety of plants and animals. Our bodies use it to activate enzymes that are important in the metabolism of glucose and fatty acids. Good sources are tea, leafy vegetables, nuts, fruits and legumes.

A healthy diet is the best insurance any man can take out if he wants to preserve his sexual energy and remain ageless and strong. So don't rely upon supplements to make up for what nature has brilliantly combined in food. Choose foods wisely and his body will reward him with a healthy, powerful physique. Now that's news you can eat!

CHAPTER 7
Why Stress Can Make Him Fat

Your man is patiently waiting for a parking spot in a crowded sports stadium when a rogue automobile comes tearing down the aisle and swings right into his slot. He hits the horn, starts screaming and vows to flatten two tires on that bozo once he finds ANOTHER spot! At that very moment he is getting fat.

You may already know that stress, especially chronic stress, taxes his heart, scrambles his brain and sabotages his immune system from working like the National Guard to protect his body against infection and cancer. Stressful situations, or even stressful thoughts, can deprive his tissue of oxygen and the chemicals necessary to keep his hormones in balance.

TO FIGHT OR FLEE:
THAT IS THE QUESTION

Just imagine your guy is a wildebeest snoozing on the Serengeti plains. Life is good and he doesn't have a care in the world. That is, until he gets a whiff of the lion that just showed up. Suddenly his heart takes the elevator to the top floor along with his blood pressure and he passes on being the blue plate special for the day and runs like hell. During those few moments, his brain faxed his adrenals to squeeze out cortisol, norepinephrine and adrenaline or epinephrine to give him the energy for this life-or-death emergency. Once he's safe, his body "stands down," and resumes its normal function. Or at least that's how his body was designed.

Unfortunately, in our high-stress society, we put ourselves through disaster training several times a day, triggering these hormones to grab high-octane fat and quick-burning glucose for energy to supply our brain, heart and muscles. And with this process come messages that tell his body that it's necessary to store even more fat. There's no question all that cortisol increases fat deposition in one place, the worst place of all...the belly.

Emotional stress is harder on a man's body than physical stress

STRESS CAN BREAK HIS HEART

Men are most certainly the more fragile of the sexes when it comes to tolerating mental stress. Just ask one of them to give a speech and his levels of epinephrine, norepinephrine and cortisol go through the roof, along with his blood pressure, while the blood flow through his heart muscle turns into that of a hundred pound weakling.[228] Men are more afraid of public speaking than death, according to researchers, which explains why most guys, when given a choice, would rather be the one in the coffin than have to deliver a eulogy.

Emotional stress is harder on a man's body than physical stress. It can increase the heart's demand for oxygen while reducing the supply of oxygen, even at low heart rates. Just being stressed can significantly increase a man's risk for a future heart attack. [229,230] More importantly, it can lower his testosterone.[231]

Anger also stresses a man's heart. While many women can vent their anger easily, many men just swallow it and maintain a hostile attitude that can change their electrocardiogram in a not-so-funny way, causing irregular heart beats and signs of cardiac oxygen starvation.[232,233] Even screaming can increase cortisol levels, which leads to artery-clogging cholesterol deposits in coronary blood vessels.[234,235]

Not surprisingly, men are great at one thing: dropping dead from heart attacks brought on by stress.[236] Frankly, males are less adaptive emotionally, physiologically and behaviorally to stress, which contributes to their increased risk for heart disease.[237]

PUTTING HIS TESTICLES IN A TWIST

Stress packs a wallop throughout his whole body and can affect his ability to produce testosterone. The hypothalamic-pituitary-gonadal (HPG) axis is his neuroendocrine switchboard, which can be jammed by proteins that inhibit enzymes necessary for testosterone production. When cortisol levels go up, they act like little bombs in his hormonal mailbox. It seems the vagus nerve, which regulates stomach acid production, begins to become extra-sensitive, releasing more norepinephrine and histamine, even when he sleeps.[238] His blood pressure starts to rise and so does his risk for a stroke and impotency.[239] And if he spends sleepless nights worrying about work, he might as well be counting pounds instead of sheep.

FATTENING UP HIS SLEEP CYCLE CAN TRIM HIS WEIGHT

You open your left eye and peek at the clock. It's 2 AM and your man is tossing and turning, keeping you awake. Since he can't get back to sleep, he turns on the TV just to hear the test pattern play white noise in the background. He feels unhappy and depressed — sort of out of sync with his life. Unfortunately, disturbances in his ability to sleep can cause both of you to gain weight.

Serotonin, that feel good hormone, is a precursor to melatonin, which is produced by the pineal gland in the brain, a pea size organ behind the hypothalamus. Melatonin helps regulate sleep.

Melatonin has other roles, and one of them is regulation of glucose by the central nervous system in a non-insulin dependent manner.[240] When he sleeps, melatonin levels go up in response to darkness and go down when his eyes are exposed to light. But if he's unable to stay asleep long enough, he can disturb the glucose levels in his blood that keep his brain fed during the night.[241] His body rhythm gets out of whack and this causes less growth hormone to be produced.

Remember, growth hormone and testosterone (estrogen in your case) mobilize fat in the body, while cortisol and insulin store fat. Growth hormone (GH) peaks during sleep just before he starts to dream, so if he isn't getting several episodes of rapid eye movement sleep (REM) in a night, he can't produce sufficient GH and melatonin to keep his blood glucose levels in check.

Tossing and turning does more than rustle the sheets. Between the ages of 25 and 35, a man can experience a 75% drop in growth hormone production if he isn't dreaming several times a night, and this translates into sustained elevated levels of cortisol.[242] Not only does that suppress testosterone production, but increased levels of cortisol may promote agitated sleep patterns.[243,244] That's not all. Sleep deprivation can lower both your metabolisms by dropping thyroid hormone levels, increase blood sugar and accelerate metabolic aging.[245] In short, you both get fat when he's stressed.

BLIND TO CANCER

Scientists notice weird things in life...and the remarkable fact that blind people have a lower incidence of hormonal-related cancers has focused science's attention upon melatonin.[246] This hormone is produced at night by a tiny gland in your brain, the pineal. Light inhibits its production. In blind people, melatonin production is never inhibited by light exposure. Living in the Arctic, where light deficit is a way of life, also seems to convey a lower risk for cancer, though I'm not ready to move from sunny California to Alaska just to enjoy the benefit.[247] But melatonin has been shown to inhibit the growth of prostate cells, whether benign or malignant.[248-250]

Just in case you thought giving him melatonin in a pill was the cure for burning the midnight oil – think again. When given in supplements, melatonin increases production of somatostatin, a hormone that turns off glucagon and growth hormone production. If this system is disturbed, it takes the rhythm of darkness and light in a 24 hour period to turn it back on. Sleep deprivation lowers his metabolism and the production of testosterone and melatonin. Several studies have looked at obesity and sleep disturbances and found that both depression and sleep alterations were signs of insulin resistance.[251-253] In particular, abdominal weight gain was confirmed by an increased waist-hip ratio due to high levels of cortisol directing fat storage to the abdomen instead of the thighs.[254] Tossing and turning all night consistently inhibits the ability of the body to produce GH-releasing hormone which tells the body to produce GH and increases the amount of insulin-like growth factor-I. Acting like a zombie may get him featured in the next Blair Witch project, but it won't help his testosterone production. The good news? Nine hours of sleep a night, and his hormones will go back to normal.[255]

DON'T HOLD HIS BREATH

Another important medical problem, sleep apnea or breath holding, can happen when he doesn't get enough sleep. Studies have shown a strong link between a Buddha Belly and sleep apnea. More significantly, sleep apnea can lead to plaques in his carotid artery and other important blood vessels, such as the ones inside the penis, making erections less strong.[256,257] It seems sleep is a very active metabolic time, and if he doesn't get enough oxygen during the night he can gain weight or turn off his weight-loss mechanism by reducing the production of growth hormone and testosterone. This changes his energy balance and insulin sensitivity creating a change in his brain's response to serotonin.[258] In a study of the relationship between lowered sympathetic nerve activity and obesity, researchers found that humans become more sensitive to essential fatty acids in their blood when serotonin levels drop and that makes us not only fat, but also depressed.[259,260]

Psychological stress makes him a target for illness

SICK AND TIRED

Long-term stress not only causes weight gain but also undermines his immune system. Men become susceptible to colds and flus and feel just plain tired. Wounds take longer to heal because cortisol prevents the normal buildup of killer white cells in the body. Even just taking a test can stress anyone out and make them sick. Dental students were given wounds to the roofs of their mouths three days before final exams and again during summer vacation (does this give you an idea of what professors think of their students?). Not surprisingly, the wounds took 40% longer to heal during test time because of a 70% decline in the production of a particular type of white blood cell messenger RNA.[261] This same response was found in caretakers of Alzheimer patients, proving that psychological stress can make you a target for illness. [262]

WHAT DID YOU SAY DEAR?

If your man has ever spent hours looking for his

checkbook, or that credit card bill that's due tomorrow, he may be experiencing memory loss from stress. Glucocorticoids, the adrenal steroid hormones secreted during stress, can damage the hippocampus or memory center of his brain by depriving the tissue of energy-producing glucose.[263] Only four hours of stress can uncouple the neurons in his brain, thanks to the plentiful receptors for corticosterone, the stress hormone in the hippocampus. This can shrivel his learning ability and may even cause brain cancer.[264] Repeated stress causes brain cells to shrink and can permanently damage nerve cells.[265] A recent study at McGill University in Quebec found that older people with high cortisol levels had smaller hippocampi and showed greater memory loss than their less-stressed peers. Stress hormones block the pituitary's ability to send signals to the testicles to produce testosterone, and these same hormones make his testicles less responsive. The net result – testosterone production is suppressed. Without testosterone, there is no control over damage from corticosterone in the brain.[266] No wonder he seems to be having a "senior moment" about those car keys.

STRESS BUSTERS

So, now that you realize how destructive stress can be in your man's life, what are you going to do about it? Here are some ideas:

- Laugh.
     It may sound silly, but laughter not only supplies oxygen to his body, it creates movement. So you have to watch old episodes of Benny Hill or The Three Stooges with him...just do it so you get him laughing again.

- Breathe.
     Meditation has garnered new attention as

researchers are confirming an association between meditation practices and levels of melatonin.[267] It can also reduce heart disease.[268] You don't have to become "Zen" to know the importance of taking in lots of oxygen for your tissue's health.

- **Pose.**

  Yoga or meditation lower stress hormones. If he is feeling stressed, show him how to assume the balance pose or T posture. Begin by standing comfortably, arms at your sides, and slowly fold forward from the hips. Extend your arms past your ears and bring your torso parallel to the ground. Simultaneously extend your left leg straight behind you. Breathe deeply and aim for stillness. Gently come back to a standing position and switch sides.

- **Exercise.**

  Don't let him exercise after 8 p.m., as this blunts production of melatonin and alters his circadian body clock.[269] Instead, help him find time during the day to get a workout. For some men, running helps them meditate in motion.

- **Walk.**

  Take 15 minutes a day for both of you to soak in the sunshine. Not only will it improve his mood, but it can also help him lose weight by adjusting his melatonin cycle and making him more responsive to insulin.[270]

- **Sleep.**

  Get to bed by 9 p.m. Melatonin levels start to rise around 9:30 so pay attention to how much light he is exposed to in a 24-hour period. At least 9 hours of sleep are required by his body to reset his biological clock and improve his insulin sensitivity. Keep naps short, around 20 minutes, in order not to reset his melatonin cycle. Trouble falling asleep? Draw him a bath. When your body normally gets ready for sleep, your temperature drops. A bath can help nudge his bedtime chemistry along. Better yet, join him in the bath for some quiet time together.

- **Inhale.**

    Pay attention to aromas. Cleopatra soaked the sails of her ship in fragrant oils to announce her approach to Rome. Try relaxing oils of ylang ylang, bergamot, tuberose, motia or orange soaked on a cotton ball. Inhaling a fragrance can stir pleasing memories which cause endorphins, the body's natural pain killers, to be released. Burn a candle or put a diffuser in the room. Just a few whiffs of lavender oil can lull you both to sleep.

- **Forgive.**

    Harboring a grudge harms his health as much as his spirit. Irritation causes the body to secrete cortisol and norepinephrine in excess, so get rid of negative emotions.

- **Pray.**

    Prayer-walking, also known as "walking meditation" provides an easy way to be active and relieve stress. It can be a meandering saunter down a garden path or a brisk march around a track. The point is to walk with prayerful intentions realizing that your journey is an interior one.

CHAPTER 8
Fueling His Fire
With Exercise

There are few ways a man can prove his virility when lying flat on his back. Hoisting metal plates at the risk of herniation may be the gold standard in gyms, but strengthening a different group of muscles can make him shine like sunlit chrome in the bedroom. But before you lose yourself in visions of steamy jungle sex, you need to understand how you can help to motivate your King Kong to exercise for his health.

Let's face it. Men enjoy getting sweaty and compete to acquire odors only wart hogs could love. So why are so few men exercising today? The answer may lie in our fast-paced lifestyle, which promotes television, remote control and beer as the trinity of a national religion. When we replace physical activity with technical advances, we become efficiency experts and the amount of energy consumed by manual labor drops. Top that off with increased stress and you have the makings of a hormonal Chernobyl.

Exercise cuts the amount of fat circulating in our bloodstreams, both immediately and long-term. Moderate exercise, especially in men, can keep cholesterol levels in check by increasing the sensitivity of fat-mobilizing enzymes to insulin.[271] Just being a couch potato nearly quadruples a man's risk of gallstones and diabetes.[272,273] And without a doubt, packing on the pounds increases vascular problems such as hypertension, heart disease and impotency.[274,275]

THE SECRET HANDSHAKE

Did you know the strength of a man's handshake at middle age can predict whether a man will be disabled by age 70? Researchers in 1965 studied hand grip strength in Japanese-American men living on Oahu, Hawaii as part of the Honolulu Heart program. When they retested these same men twenty five years later, the risk of being disabled and needing assistance living was more than twice as great in those with the lowest hand grip strength when compared to men with fists of steel. It's no secret that good muscle strength may protect men from old age disability.[276]

THE CHALLENGE

A man needs challenges and rewards to convince him to exercise. No amount of nagging or prodding can take the place of the personal realization that he can regain control of his body and his life by following the Gladiator Diet lifestyle. So, I'm not going to discuss all the exercises a man can do to gain muscle strength. Other books and even magazines can do a far better job than I, and I've listed some excellent sources in Appendix A. But I will share with you the effect certain sports and exercises can have on your Hercules' ability to make you sing the praises of Zeus in bed. After all, if your Greek god is not in physical shape, sex can kill him.[277]

BENT ON RIDING

With the current federal mandate to "double non motorized transportation," bicycling offers the potential for cleaner air, healthier people and better use of precious road space. However, new studies point the finger at seat design in causing damage to a man's urethra, prostate and the blood supply to his penis. It seems all that compression can seriously hurt the small arteries that pump blood into the corporal bodies of the penis, resulting in impotency in otherwise healthy individuals.[278] The person at greatest risk...the weekend rider. And this is not an isolated study. Measurements of prostate-specific antigen, or PSA (which gives an index of prostate health), were more elevated after bicycle riding in men with enlarged prostates.[279] He can increase blood flow simply by changing position often and shifting between resting on the seat and standing on the pedals.[280]

New seat designs that put less pressure on his prostate are one answer, but here's another idea. Suggest he try a "bent" or recumbent bike. It's the most fun I've ever had in a horizontal position. Okay, so I'm lying. With an estimated 15,000 recumbents sold in 1998 alone, these bikes are becoming a serious mainstream alternative for men who want a comfortable, prostate-safe mode of transportation. Think of it as taking a spin on a Barcalounger but without the dorky looks.

What makes the ride so great? The special cantilevered fork on the load-bearing rear wheel acts as a shock absorber and the seat cushion is padded with a great back support. Your biker can pedal longer without tiring, which helps him burn more fat. His butt will shape up too because recumbent bikes do more for his hamstrings and glutes. As for other body parts, cycling in the recumbent position puts less weight on his wrists, knees, shoulders and neck.

If your man is like me, crashing can be a hazard to one's health. The good news? You run into objects feet first. This can be a benefit, since bikers sustain an alarmingly high injury rate, according to the 1998 U.S. Consumer Product Safety Commission's report. With a shape like a low rider, don't be surprised if he begs you to get him one. Just ignore the whimpering.

KICKBOXING

Mention Bruce Lee or "Enter the Dragon" and most men happily begin flailing their arms about like a ninja turtle on speed. Cardio-kickboxing, or boxing aerobics, is a hybrid of boxing, martial arts and aerobic dance that offers a high-intensity, aggression-releasing workout without the mind-numbing boredom of other spandex challenged endeavors. Men who exercise this way can expect to burn 350 to 450 calories per hour while maintaining a heart rate at 75 to 80 percent of maximum, much like an hour of brisk walking or light jogging. However, all this testosterone dumping comes with a significant risk of injury. Elbows, shoulders, knees and backs, not to mention strained groin muscles, top the list of damages that can be done when his form is not "prize fight" ready. So do him a favor and get a beginner's video for him to watch and train with before taking on classes at a gym, where instructors teach to the more advanced people in the class. By minimizing his risk of injury, you'll be the only one to judge whether he's a "contender" in your ring at night.

RUN BABY RUN

If ever there was a sport in which men were anatomically designed to excel, it's running. Men's pelvic floors don't need to "birth no babies". Instead, they were given a tighter, narrower outlet of muscles which can act like a trampoline whenever bowels bounce against them. Running can also protect a man against disability and even death. In a study performed over eight years, members of running clubs not only had a much lower incidence of disability, but lived longer than those who didn't exercise aerobically.[281]

However, strenuous exercise can cause blood to appear in his urine, especially after biking or running.

Known as "runner's hematuria" it most often is due to bruising of the bladder neck, where delicate blood vessels can become overloaded and congested. A diet without enough protein contributes to this benign syndrome.[282] Just resting makes the blood disappear, but if it persists, send your man to a urologist.

IMPROVE THE FLOW

Want to increase blood flow to his penis? Suggest he do a few leg presses at the gym. Just 30 seconds after a man presses around 75% of his maximum exercising weight, blood flow to the tip of the penis increases more than 21%.[280] That means more oxygen is available to get into the power cells that keep the penis hard as a diamond cutter...and we know how much ladies love diamonds! Remember, a firm, hard

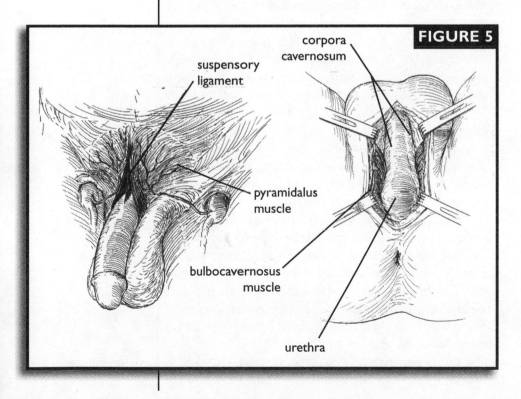

FIGURE 5

corpora cavernosum

suspensory ligament

pyramidalus muscle

bulbocavernosus muscle

urethra

erection depends on a healthy blood flow into two chambers in his penis, called corpora cavernosa, through the mesh network of blood vessels, or corpora spongiosum. (Figure 5) Amazingly, an erect penis can hold eight times as much blood as a flaccid one, which explains why men have such difficulty thinking during sex.

PENIS PUSHUPS

Men worry about angles. It's a fact that as they age, the angle of their erections drops from something on which you could hang a paint bucket to something that looks more useful for stirring the paint. Even with a full erection, men over 50 discover they can't snap their penis against their abdomen like they used to! The muscle responsible for this feat is the bulbocavernosus, a thick, spoon-shaped muscle that supports the urethra and is responsible for shooting sperm like a cannonball out of the penis during orgasm. In conjunction with the levator ani, a sling of muscles that make up the pelvic floor, and the pyramidalis muscle on the abdominal wall, these "sex machines" help increase pressure within the chambers of the penis, giving a fuller erection. However, as testosterone levels drop, so does the strength of these muscles. Having performed numerous penile implants during my residency, I can attest first-hand to this observation.

But all is not lost with age. Much as women need to practice tightening their pelvic floor muscles to prevent minor accidents when sneezing, men should perform daily "penis pushups" to keep the "angle of the dangle" as high as possible. This is not just vanity...as the higher the angle of his penis, the better his glans can massage your "G" spot during intercourse. As you saw in Chapter 7, the addition of low-dose testosterone can greatly strengthen these muscles. But let me share with you the best way to get him to perform this exercise.

Have him begin practicing his pushups early in the morning, when he has an erection from a full bladder. Place the palm of your hand above his penis. Have him tighten his anal sphincter and contract, while lifting his abdominal muscles. This will bring his penis up against the palm of your hand. Then have him relax. Repeat this 10 times, gradually working up to a count of 30. His reward?... a fuller erection. Now assume your favorite position for sex (the Trojan horse perhaps?) and after penetration you'll contract your pelvic floor muscles together, which should intensify the sensation for both of you. Inevitably, this leads to all-out get-down jungle sex as you find a new rhythm to your beat. Keep practicing and the two of you could end up on a Wheaties box. I can guarantee you he won't miss a single session!

This exercise plan, however, does come with a warning:

1) Do not attempt to perform push ups at red lights or while wearing constrictive clothing.

2) If performed while brushing one's teeth, step back from the cabinet edge to avoid injury.

3) Do not attempt to operate machinery while performing this exercise.

4) Do not attempt to perform this exercise while urinating. Damage to bathroom walls is not covered under the warranty and will void any future use of your penis for 72 hours.

CHAPTER 9
Staying the Championship Course

Trust me. This next step won't hurt one little bit. All you need is a tape measure to start him off on his own personal journey to a slimmer, more virile body. So let's get started.

CALCULATING BODY MASS INDEX

Remember that weight is not the factor which indicates how healthy your warrior is, but rather three measurements: Body Mass Index, waist circumference and percent body fat. It's easy to measure his waistline — no tickling now! Just place the tape around the smallest part of his abdomen above his belly button and below his lowest rib. Go to the chart on the next page and write down his waistline in inches. The next two figures are a bit more complicated. To determine his Body Mass Index, you need to take his height and convert it into inches and then meters squared. The chart makes it easier. Now have him go weigh himself. Don't worry. Tell him you won't look.

I've included detailed instructions in the chart to help you complete his profile. To determine his percent body fat, I highly recommend the new electronic scale by Tanita or the hand-held device by Omron. Both devices emit a low electrical current that calculates both the percent and actual pounds of fat on his body. Skin calipers can also give him an accurate reading. The gold standard involves submersion in water to determine the precise amount of body fat. But if your man is "water soluble" he'll prefer the electronic scale readings to keep track of his progress.

Now, if you want to know his basal metabolic rate or BMR (how many calories he burns just sitting) multiply his weight in pounds by 11. This will give you a rough idea of how many 350-calorie meals he needs in a day just to keep breathing. Now add 350 calories for walking, fidgeting or fixing the car and you have how many calories he needs to maintain his current weight. Once you are armed with this information, you are ready to proceed to the next step.

	21	22	23	24	25	26	27	28	29	30
5'2"	115	120	126	131	136	142	147	153	158	164
5'3"	118	124	130	135	141	146	152	158	163	169
5'4"	122	128	134	140	145	151	157	163	169	174
5'5"	126	132	138	144	150	156	162	168	174	180
5'6"	130	136	142	148	155	161	167	173	179	186
5'7"	134	140	146	153	159	166	172	178	185	191
5'8"	138	144	151	158	164	171	177	184	190	197
5'9"	142	149	155	162	169	176	182	189	196	203
5'10"	146	153	160	167	174	181	188	195	202	207
5'11"	150	157	165	172	179	186	193	200	208	215
6'0"	155	160	170	175	185	190	200	205	215	220
6'1"	160	165	175	180	190	195	205	210	220	225
6'2"	160	170	180	185	195	200	210	215	225	230

To calculate body mass index:

1. Waist   _____inches
                        Goal: Under 30 inches

2. Height   _____inches
                        (multiply feet by 12 and add the rest as inches)

_____ meters^2 To convert to meters, multiply inches by 0.0254 then multiply that number against itself

Example 62 inches x 0.0254 =1.5748 x 1.5748=2.479 meters^2

3. Weight   _____pounds (To convert to kilograms, divide by 2.2)
                                _____kg

4. $BMI = kg/m2$ _____ Simply take #3 divided by #2
                         Goal: Under 25 kg/m2

5. Percent body fat _____
                         Goal: Under 15%

6. BMR =   _____ calories
                        (weight in pounds x 11)

Calories/350 =   _____ mini meals/day

To lose weight, simply add 350 calories of exercise and drop out one macho meal a day.

THE FAMILY TREE

I always asked my patients about risk factors hiding in their family tree, specifically what illnesses occurred and the cause of any family member's death. More than 3,000 ailments are known to be inherited, including heart disease, cancer, diabetes, arthritis, Alzheimer's, even alcoholism, depression, thyroid disease and schizophrenia. Take time to fill this form out for both sides of your family and make copies for your children. It will make his motivation even stronger for losing weight and staying healthy.

OLD MOTHER HUBBARD

Remove temptation, in the form of high glycemic carbohydrates, from your shelves. There is no truth to the rumor that calories are afraid of heights and will leap out of food if stored on the top shelf. Go on...just throw them away.

•   Designate a specific cupboard just for his own food items and place any cereals or bread in another cupboard for your family to use.

•   Replace cooking oils with olive oil, canola and peanut oil.

•   Stock up on spices and teas and get rid of cans of vegetables you've been saving since the beginning of the world.

•   Check labels for corn syrup or MSG and toss products that have them.

Once you've got this situation in hand, let's deal with the shopping list.

YOUR FAMILY HEALTH HISTORY

This blank genogram has room for only your own family history. But you can photo copy the page, add your spouse's family, and combine the two for your children's full health history. Squeeze in extra names, of course, if you have an especially large family. When your genogram is complete, give your doctor a copy for your medical files and make separate copies for your spouse's and children's files. Store another copy for each of your children and update it periodically.

Name of person submitting genogram ————————————————————

Date ————————————————————————————————————

Address ——————————————————————————————————

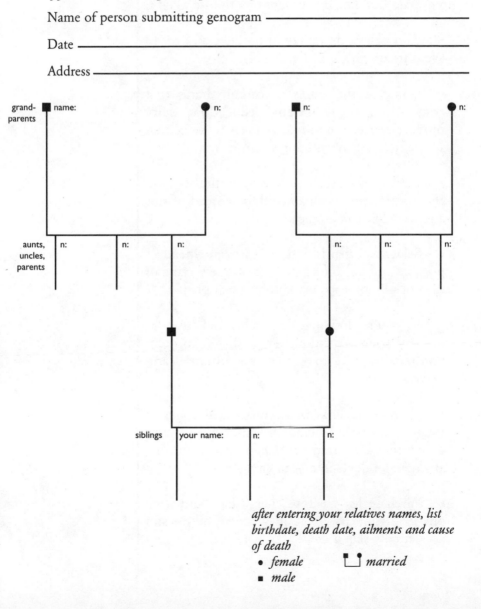

after entering your relatives names, list birthdate, death date, ailments and cause of death

- *female*   ⌐⌐ *married*
- *male*

TO MARKET TO MARKET

Copy the list of high glycemic carbohydrates on page 43 and take the list with you to the grocery store. It's important in starting The Gladiator Diet that you understand which carbohydrates have the ability to raise his blood sugar higher than the Empire State Building if you want him to lose weight.

• Choose a wide variety of produce and try to avoid frozen or canned vegetables.

• Compare the grams of carbohydrates that come from sugar in any reduced-fat dairy products versus the full fat versions to be certain you're not just substituting sugar for fat.

• Lean meats usually come from the loin, so choose filet, pork loin and sirloin instead of ribs and heavily marbled meats.

• Select fish that is fresh, not frozen whenever possible and try to include at least one serving of tuna or salmon each week in his meal plan.

• If you're looking for additional non-fat protein sources, buy whey and soy protein powders to add to soups, mayonnaise and dressings.

• Corn syrup lurks in an amazing number of soups and drinks, including some orange juice concentrates, so read the labels before putting any new products into your cart.

• Purchase low-fructose energy bars and keep one in his lunch box at all times so he doesn't accidentally skip a meal.

EATING OUT

Portion control is probably the hardest part of eating out, with today's restaurants vying to win the Gordita Grande award when it comes to a main course. The simplest way for him to overcome this is to order two appetizers and request steamed vegetables as a side dish. Include a salad but pass on the bread. Treat him to the most appetizing dessert on the menu. Remember, the composition of his previous meal affects his next one, so don't be afraid to let him make an occasional withdrawal on that carbohydrate account.

URGE TO SPLURGE

He's been great on The Gladiator Diet but he's dying for some rice or bread. Can he eat it? Of course. He can do anything he wants. But here is how to deal with the occasional craving. Prepare as much of the food as his eyes told you he wants, then put the entire serving on his plate along with his protein, fat and low glycemic carbs. Only allow him one high glycemic food at a meal every three days. After a few mouthfuls he won't need any more to satisfy his urge to splurge. So don't deny him any food on the shopping list if he has a craving for it. Just remind him – each time he eats a high glycemic carb it's like guzzling corn syrup.

CHARTING HIS PROGRESS

I recommend he weigh in once a week at the same time of day and take an inventory of his waistline every week. Notice how his clothes fit, instead of where the needle on the scale is bouncing. It's a much better indicator of losing fat. Write down his weekly values and compare them after one month. I think you'll both be pleased with the results he's achieved by not starving or denying himself.

A FINAL WORD

The ability to remain naturally strong, ageless and healthy is within the practical reach of any man. By using the principles in The Gladiator Diet Plan, he can regain the vitality and physique of his youth without the need for pills or surgery. There's no battle involved in becoming a gladiator...just a realization that low protein, high carbohydrate, non-fat diets make men age faster by increasing the risk of damage to their bodies from uncontrolled blood sugar that can lead to impotence, heart disease, strokes and cancer. So, celebrate his new look, as the song says by... "do a little (victory) dance, make a little love......" and get down with your gladiator tonight!

APPENDIX A
Resources
For Living

THE GLADIATOR DIET WEBSITE

If you are interested in learning more about the impact of diet on men's health, visit my website at

www.gladiatordiet.com

where you will find up to date news articles, discussions about the latest scientific research, and a free online newsletter, "Larrian Reports." You can order personally autographed copies of

"The Gladiator Diet" or any of my other books.

by calling

1-800-554-3335

in the United States or 310 471-2375 if you do not have access to the internet.

Don't miss out on my books for women, "The Goddess Diet" (for premenopausal women), and "The Menopause Diet", for those interested in the impact of diet and hormone therapy on their health. The Goddess Diet book contains all the same information found in The Menopause Diet and The Menopause Diet Mini Meal Cookbook, but is missing the chapter on hormone therapy. This book is intended for women who run screaming from the room at the mere mention of the "M" word, but want information that is crucial to their understanding of how our bodies change as our hormones get out of balance. The print type is smaller than in The Menopause Diet, which is designed for fearless women who prefer reading without their glasses and who already understand the power that comes with menopause. The Menopause Diet suits today's woman seeking to regain the shape and vitality of her youth without the need for pills or surgery. The 7 day menu planner is contained in The Menopause Diet Mini Meal Cookbook and incorporates the recipes in the book.

BODY FAT MONITORS

The Tanita Body Fat Monitor/Scale is available at Macy's and other large department stores. The scale measures both weight and body fat in 30 seconds and is programmable for up to four people. It retails for $149.95.

Omron makes a portable hand held body fat analyzer that works on the same principle as the Tanita model. It retails for $129.95 at The Sharper Image and several other electronic stores.

Call 1-800-634-4350 for a distributor near you.

SPICES

Purchasing new, exotic spices can lend a real zip to foods while keeping the fat low. One of the best sources is Penzeys Spice catalog. You can order their catalog on line at:

- Penzeys Spices
  www.penzeys.com
  414 679-7207

For Allepo, pasilla and ancho chili powder, Dean and Deluca is an excellent resource. You can order online at:

- Dean and Deluca
  www.dean-deluca-napavalley.com
  707 967-9880.

Other sources for exotic spices are:

- Kalustyan
  123 Lexington Ave
  New York, NY 10016
  (212) 685-3451

- Sultan's Delight
  P.O. Box 090302
  Brooklyn, NY 11209
  (800) 852-6844
  (718) 745-6844
  Fax (718) 745-2563

- The Spice House
  1031 N. Old World Third St
  Milwaukee, WI 53203
  (414) 272-0977

- Uwajimaya
  (800) 889-1928.

An excellent source for asian spices, such as chinese brown bean paste, star anise, fish sauce, chili paste.

- Foods of India
  (212) 683-4419.

Sadaf brand pomegranate paste for Middle Eastern dishes

- Chile Today—Hot Tamale
  (800) 468-7377.
  Dried New Mexican red chilis

- Kitchen Market
  (212) 243-4433.
  A great source for banana leaves and dried ancho chilis if you don't have a Latino shop nearby.

- Adriana's Caravan
  409 Vanderbilt St
  Brooklyn, NY 11218
  (718) 436-8565.
  This store will ship fresh curry leaves, tamarind concentrate, dried pomegranate seeds and brown mustard seeds.

- Frieda's
  P.O. Box 58488
  Los Angeles, Calif. 90058
  (800)-241-1771
  http://www.friedas.com
  Kaboucha squash, chilis and wax peppers can be found at this unique supplier.

TEAS

One of my favorite teas is made by Bernardaud's of France. It's a caramel tea and is rich in flavor, even when laced with a little milk. You can order it from:

- La Cucina Rustica
  cyberbaskets.com/cbdocs/items/be9003c.htm
  9950 West Lawrence Avenue, Suite 202
  Schiller Park, IL 60176 USA
  800 796-0116 — Customer Service Department

- Stash makes a Mango Passion Fruit tea available in grocery stores and Ceylon Passion has a delightful Passion Fruit Papaya tea combination. A mixture of black teas with fruit extract, they make delightful iced teas. All are caffeine free and available in your grocery store.

• Tejava is a delicious micro brewed tea made entirely from the top leaves of each branch picked only from May through October. If you can't find it in your grocery store, call 1-800-4-GEYSER

TOMATOES

There is nothing better than fresh tomatoes, but the organic canned tomatoes seasoned with sea salt by Muir Glen do well in a pinch. If you don't find them in your grocery store, call or write

• Muir Glen
  P.O. Box 1498
  Sacramento, California
  707 778-7801
  www.muirglen.com
  has a store locator on the site

SEA SALT

Searching for specialty sea salts has become a hobby of mine and I will share with you my secret sources.

• The Baker's Catalogue
  P.O. Box 876 Norwich, VT 05055-0876
  800 827-6836
  http://www.kingarthurflour.com
This company sells Maldon Crystal sea salt, Celtic Grey and Fleur de sel de Guerande, the most expensive type of salt, harvested under special conditions.

- Zingerman's
  422 Detroit St.
  Ann Arbor, MI 48104
  888 636-8162

This is another source for Fleur de sel de Guerande.

- Corti Brothers
  5810 Folsom Blvd.
  Sacramento, Calif 95822
  800 509-FOOD

This company carries Sicilian sea salt and Japanese Oshima Island salt.

THE GREATEST GRATER

Microplane has found a new use for a woodworker's rasp – zesting citrus, cheese and chocolate. These blades come in fine or coarse ratings which can be simply changed out as needed. You can purchase them from Sur La Table or from Microplane for under $15.

- Microplane Lee Valley Tools
  800 871-8158
  http://www.microplane.com

JAPANESE MANDOLINE

This nifty little device is like an apple corer only standing upright. It can make oodles of noodles out of any hard vegetable with just a turn of the handle. You can purchase one from Sur La Table.

- Sur La Table
  800 221-5786

RECUMBENT BIKES

To find a distributor for the BikeE CT 2.0, call:

- BikeE
  1-800-231-3136
  5125 S W Hout
  Corvallis, Oregon 97333
  It retails for $650.

PILATES®

If you're looking for books, videos and equipment in order to perform Pilates® contact:

- Current Concepts
  1-800-240-3539
  They have several books available. Be sure and ask for this one:

- *Body Control Pilates*
  by Lynne Robinson and Gordon Thomson
  BainBridge Books, 1998

Here are other resources for this exercise program:

- PhysicalMind Institute
  1-800-505-1990

- Pilates Studio
  1-800-474-5283
  www.pilates-studio.com
  They sell a foldable home exercise reformer for stretching

To get started on exercising, just go to any bookstore and stand in front of the health and fitness section. I recommend the following books for their clean, simple approach to understanding weight training and body shaping.

- *Body Shaping*
  by Michael Yessis, PhD.,
  Rodale Press, 1994

- *Callanetics*
  by Callan Pinckney,
  Perigee Books, 1997

- *Power Yoga*
  by Beryl Bender Birch,
  Fireside, 1995 l

If you are interested in reading about the health benefits of arginine, pick up this book:

- *The Arginine Solution*
  by Robert Fried Ph.D.
  and Woodson Merrell, MD.,
  Warner Books, 1999

There is only one book every person who has ever suffered from kidney stones should have in their home health library. It's even recommended by Former Surgeon General C. Everett Koop:

- *The Kidney Stones Handbook*,
  Gail Savitz and Stephen Leslie, M.D.,
  Four Geez Press, 1999
  1-800-2kidney
  916 781-3440
  1911 Douglass Blvd #85
  Roseville, Ca 95661

This book by Mary Shomon, About.com Thyroid Guide, will open your eyes to the effect thyroid problems can have on weight gain, depression and fatigue. Told from her own personal experience as a patient.

- *Living Well With Hypothyroidism*
  by Mary Shomon
  HarperCollins/Avon/WholeCare, 2000
  http://www.thyroid-info.com/booktoc.htm

If you want to see the full listing of foods tested to date and their GI ratings, read this book:

- *The Glucose Revolution: The Authoritative Guide to the Glycemic Index*
  by Jennie Brand Miller, Thomas Wolever and and Kaye Foster-Powell
  Marlowe & Co., 1999

If you want to try Prayer-walking, read this book:

- *The Complete Guide to Prayer-Walking*
  by Linus Mundy
  Crossroads Publications, 1997

These books on breathing will give you a practical guide to deep relaxation and much more:

- *The Breathing Book*
  by Donna Farhi,
  Owl Books, 1996

- *The Tao of Natural Breathing*
  by Dennis Lewis,
  Mountain Wind Publishing, 1997

- *Conscious Breathing*
  by Gay Hendricks, Ph.D.,
  Bantam Books, 1995

MAGAZINES

There are numerous men's health magazines that focus on exercise techniques for men. Give your man a subscription to any of the following:

- Men's Health
- Men's Fitness
- Muscular Development
- Muscle and Fitness

APPENDIX B
References

1. Mokdad, A.H., *et al.*, *The spread of the obesity epidemic in the United States, 1991-1998.* Jama, 1999. **282**(16): p. 1519-22.

2. Everett, J., *et al.*, *Special Report The Average Man Survey*, in Men's Health. 2000. p. 59-68.

3. Rimm, E., *et al. Body weight, physical activity, and alcohol consumption in relation to erectile dysfunction among US male health professionals free of major chronic diseases.* in American Urologic Association. 2000. Atlanta, Georgia: Journal of Urology.

4. Bjorntorp, P., *The regulation of adipose tissue distribution in humans.* Int J Obes Relat Metab Disord, 1996. **20**(4): p. 291-302.

5. Strain, G.W., *et al.*, *Effect of massive weight loss on hypothalamic-pituitary-gonadal function in obese men.* J Clin Endocrinol Metab, 1988. **66**(5): p. 1019-23.

6. Lotufo, P.A., *et al.*, *Male pattern baldness and coronary heart disease: the Physicians' Health Study.* Arch Intern Med, 2000. **160**(2): p. 165-71.

7. English, K.M., *et al.*, *Men with coronary artery disease have lower levels of androgens than men with normal coronary angiograms [In Process Citation].* Eur Heart J, 2000. **21**(11): p. 890-4.

8. Johannes, C.B., *et al.*, *Incidence of erectile dysfunction in men 40 to 69 years old: longitudinal results from the Massachusetts male aging study [see comments].* J Urol, 2000. **163**(2): p. 460-3.

9. Wilson, J. and D. Foster, Williams Textbook of Endocrinology. 8 ed. 1992, Philadelphia: W.B. Saunders.

10. Marin, P. and S. Arver, *Androgens and abdominal obesity.* Baillieres Clin Endocrinol Metab, 1998. **12**(3): p. 441-51.

11. Gambineri, A. and R. Pasquali, *Testosterone therapy in men: clinical and pharmacological perspectives [In Process Citation].* J Endocrinol Invest, 2000. **23**(3): p. 196-214.

12. Lam, W.F., *et al.*, *Influence of hyperglycemia on the satiating effect*

of CCK in humans [In Process Citation]. Physiol Behav, 1998. **65**(3): p. 505-11.

13. Longcope, C., *et al.*, *Diet and sex hormone binding globulin.* J Clin Endocrinol Metab, 2000. **85**(1): p. 293-6.

14. Marquis, J., *Most Californians Are Fat, Study Finds,* in Los Angeles Times. 2000: Los Angeles. p. A3,26.

15. Gensini, G.F., M. Comeglio, and A. Colella, *Classical risk factors and emerging elements in the risk profile for coronary artery disease.* Eur Heart J, 1998. 19 Suppl A: p. A53-61.

16. Anate, M., A. Olatinwo, and A. Omesina, *Obesity—an overview.* West Afr J Med, 1998. **17**(4): p. 248-54.

17. Large, V. and P. Arner, *Regulation of lypolysis in humans. Pathophysiological modulation in obesity, diabetes and hyperlipidaemia.* Diabetes Metab, 1998. **24**(5): p. 409-18.

18. Maurer, K.R., *et al.*, *Risk factors for gallstone disease in the Hispanic populations of the United States.* Am J Epidemiol, 1990. **131**(5): p. 836-44.

19. Curhan, G.C., *et al.*, *Body size and risk of kidney stones.* J Am Soc Nephrol, 1998. **9**(9): p. 1645-52.

20. Carey, D.G., *et al.*, *Abdominal fat and insulin resistance in normal and overweight women: Direct measurements reveal a strong relationship in subjects at both low and high risk of NIDDM.* Diabetes, 1996. **45**(5): p. 633-8.

21. Goldsmith, H., The Omentum. 1990, New York: Springer-Verlag.

22. Bronnegard, M., *et al.*, *Glucocorticoid receptor messenger ribonucleic acid in different regions of human adipose tissue.* Endocrinology, 1990. **127**(4): p. 1689-96.

23. Iannoli, P., *et al.*, *Glucocorticoids upregulate intestinal nutrient transport in a time-dependent and substrate-specific fashion.* Gastrointest Surg, 1998. **2**(5): p. 449-57.

24. Bjorntorp, P., *Metabolic difference between visceral and subcutaneous abdominal fat.* Diabetes Metab, 2000. **26**(3): p. 10-12.

25. Andersson, S.O., *et al.*, *Body size and prostate cancer: a 20-year follow-up study among 135006 Swedish construction workers.* J Natl Cancer Inst, 1997. **89**(5): p. 385-9.

26. Fraumeni, J.F., Jr., *Cancers of the pancreas and biliary tract: epidemiological considerations.* Cancer Res, 1975. **35**(11 Pt. 2): p. 3437-46.

27. Barbieri, R., *Adipose Tissue and Reproduction.* Prog Reprod Biol Med, ed. R. Frisch. Vol. 14. 1990, Basel: Karger. 42-57.

28. Lemieux, S., *et al.*, *A single threshold value of waist girth identifies normal-weight and overweight subjects with excess visceral adipose tissue.* Am J Clin Nutr, 1996. **64**: p. 685-93.

29. Ruderman, N., *et al.*, *The metabolically obese, normal-weight individual revisited.* Diabetes, 1998. **47**(5): p. 699-713.

30. Lyu, L.C., *et al.*, *Relationship of body fat distribution with cardiovascular risk factors in healthy Chinese.* Ann Epidemiol, 1994. **4**(6): p. 434-44.

31. De Pergola, G., *et al.*, *Lower androgenicity is associated with higher plasma levels of prothrombotic factors irrespective of age, obesity, body fat distribution, and related metabolic parameters in men.* Metabolism, 1997. **46**(11): p. 1287-93.

32. Donahue, R.P., *et al.*, *Central obesity and coronary heart disease in men.* Lancet, 1987. **1**(8537): p. 821-4.

33. Ashwell, M., *Obesity in men and women [see comments].* Int J Obes Relat Metab Disord, 1994. **18** Suppl 1: p. S1-7.

34. Harris, M., *Epidemiological correlates of NIDDM in Hispanics, whites and blacks in the US population.* Diabetes Care, 1991. **14**(Suppl 3): p. S639-S648.

35. Gavin, J., *The role of the gastrointestinal tract and alpha-glucosidase inhibition in Type II diabetes.* Drug Benefits Trends, 1996 (Supp 8E): p. 18-26.

36. Jarrett, R., H. Keen, and J.Fulley, *et al.,Worsening to diabetes in men with impaired glucose tolerance (borderline diabetes).* Diabetologia, 1979. 16: p. 25-30.

37. Yarnell, J.W., *et al.*, *Comparison of weight in middle age, weight at 18 years, and weight change between, in predicting subsequent 14 year mortality and coronary events: caerphilly prospective study [In Process Citation].* J Epidemiol Community Health, 2000. **54**(5): p. 344-8.

38. Grivetti, L.E. and E.A. Applegate, *From Olympia to Atlanta: a cultural-historical perspective on diet and athletic training.* J Nutr, 1997. **127**(5 Suppl): p. 860S-868S.

39. Coakley, E.H., *et al.*, *Predictors of weight change in men: results from the Health Professionals Follow-up Study.* Int J Obes Relat Metab Disord, 1998. **22**(2): p. 89-96.

40. Raskin, P., *et al.*, *Abnormal alpha cell function in human diabetes: the response to oral protein.* Am J Med, 1978. **64**(6): p. 988-97.

41. Wagner, R. and J. Warkany, *Untersuchungen uber den zuckerbildenden Wert der Gemuse in der Diabetikerkost.* Z Kinderheilk, 1927. 44: p. 322.

42. Crapo, P., G. Reaven, and J. Olefsky, *Plasma glucose and insulin*

responses to orally administered simple and complex carbohydrates. Diabetes, 1976. 25: p. 741-747.

43.   Wolever, T.M., *et al., Glycemic index of foods in individual subjects.* Diabetes Care, 1990. **13**(2): p. 126-32.

44.   Jenkins, D., T. Wolever, and R. Taylor, *Glycemic index of foods: a physiological basis for carbohydrate exchange.* Am J Clin Nutr, 1981. 34: p. 362-6.

45.   Juliano, B.O., *et al., Properties of Thai cooked rice and noodles differing in glycemic index in noninsulin-dependent diabetics [published erratum appears in Plant Foods Hum Nutr 1990 Jul;40(3):231-2].* Plant Foods Hum Nutr, 1989. **39**(4): p. 369-74.

46.   Wolever, T., *et al., Glycaemic index of 102 complex carbohydrate foods in patients with diabetes.* Nutr Res, 1994. 14: p. 651-669.

47.   Nuttall, F., *et al., Effect of protein ingestion on the glucose and insulin response to a standardized oral glucose load.* Diabetes Care, 1984. 7: p. 465-470.

48.   Smith, G.P. and J. Gibbs, *Are gut peptides a new class of anorectic agents?* Am J Clin Nutr, 1992. **55**(1 Suppl): p. 283S-285S.

49.   Welch, I., *et al., Duodenal and ileal lipid suppresses postprandial blood glucose an dinsulin responses in man: possible implications for the dietary managment of diabetes mellitus.* Clin Sci, 1987. 72: p. 209-216.

50.   Collier, G., T. Wolever, and D. Jenkins, *Concurrent ingestion of fat and reduction in starch content impairs carbohydrate tolerance to subsequent meals.* Am J Clin Nutr, 1987. 45: p. 963-969.

51.   Wolever, T.M. and C. Bolognesi, *Prediction of glucose and insulin responses of normal subjects after consuming mixed meals varying in energy, protein, fat, carbohydrate and glycemic index.* J Nutr, 1996. **126**(11): p. 2807-12.

52.   Jenkins, D., *et al., Metabolic effects of a low-glycemic-index diet.* Am J Clin Nutr, 1987. **46**(6): p. 968-75.

53.   Jenkins, D., T. Wolever, and G. Buckley, *et al., Low glycemic index starchy foods in the diabetic diet.* AM J Clin Nutr, 1988. 48: p. 248-254.

54.   LeBlanc, J., I. Mercier, and A. Nadeau, *Components of postprandial thermogenesis in relation to meal frequency in humans.* Can J Physiol Pharmacol, 1993. **71**(12): p. 879-83.

55.   Jenkins, D., *et al., "Nibbling versus gorging": metabolic advantages of increased meal frequency.* N Eng J Med, 1989. 321: p. 929-34.

56.   Jenkins, D.J., *et al., Low glycemic index: lente carbohydrates and physiological effects of altered food frequency.* Am J Clin Nutr, 1994. **59**(3 Suppl): p. 706S-709S.

57. LeBlanc, J. and J. *Soucy, Interactions between post-prandial thermogenesis, sensory stimulation of feeding, and hunger.* Am J Physiol, 1996. **271**(4 Pt 2): p. R936-40.

58. Soucy, J. and J. Leblanc, *Protein meals and postprandial thermogenesis.* Physiol Behav, 1999. **65**(4-5): p. 705-9.

59. Leibowitz, S.F., A. Akabayashi, and J. Wang, *Obesity on a high-fat diet: role of hypothalamic galanin in neurons of the anterior paraventricular nucleus projecting to the median eminence.* J Neurosci, 1998. **18**(7): p. 2709-19.

60. Himaya, A. and J. Louis-Sylvestre, *The effect of soup on satiation.* Appetite, 1998. **30**(2): p. 199-210.

61. Wolever, T.M., *et al., Second-meal effect: low-glycemic-index foods eaten at dinner improve subsequent breakfast glycemic response.* Am J Clin Nutr, 1988. **48**(4): p. 1041-7.

62. Parodi, P.W., *The French paradox unmasked: the role of folate.* Med Hypotheses, 1997. **49**(4): p. 313-8.

63. Chatenoud, L., *et al., Whole grain food intake and cancer risk.* Int J Cancer, 1998. **77**(1): p. 24-8.

64. La Vecchia, C. and A. Tavani, *Fruit and vegetables, and human cancer.* Eur J Cancer Prev, 1998. **7**(1): p. 3-8.

65. Monneuse, M.O., F. Bellisle, and G. Koppert, *Eating habits, food and health related attitudes and beliefs reported by French students.* Eur J Clin Nutr, 1997. **51**(1): p. 46-53.

66. Larson, D.E., *et al., Dietary fat in relation to body fat and intraabdominal adipose tissue: a cross-sectional analysis [see comments].* Am J Clin Nutr, 1996. **64**(5): p. 677- 84.

67. Ginsberg, H.N., *et al., Effects of reducing dietary saturated fatty acids on plasma lipids and lipoproteins in healthy subjects: the DELTA Study, protocol 1.* Arterioscler Thromb Vasc Biol, 1998. **18**(3): p. 441-9.

68. Low, C., E. Grossman, and B. Gumbiner, *Potentiation of effects of weight loss by monunsaturated fatty acids in obese NIDDM patients.* Diabetes, 1996. 45: p. 569-575.

69. O'Byrne, D.J., D.A. Knauft, and R.B. Shireman, *Low fat-monounsaturated rich diets containing high-oleic peanuts improve serum lipoprotein profiles.* Lipids, 1997. **32**(7): p. 687-95.

70. Trautwein, E.A., *et al., Effect of dietary fats rich in lauric, myristic, palmitic, oleic or linoleic acid on plasma, hepatic and biliary lipids in cholesterol-fed hamsters.* Br J Nutr, 1997. **77**(4): p. 605-20.

71. Agriculture, U.S.D.A., USDA Food Guide Pyramid. 1996.

72. Grundy, S., *Comparison of monounsaturated fatty acids and carbohydrates for lowering plasma cholesterol.* N Eng J Med, 1986. 314: p. 745-748.

73. Garg, A., *et al., Comparison of a high-carbohydrate diet with a high-monounsaturated-fat diet in patients with non-insulin-dependent diabetes mellitus.* N Engl J Med, 1988. **319**(13): p. 829-34.

74. Brunner, D., J. Weisbort, and N. Meshulam, *et al., Relation of serum total cholesterol and high-density lipoprotein cholesterol percentage to the incidence of definite coronary events:twenty-year follow-up of the Donolo-Tel Aviv prospetive coronary artery disease study.* Am J Cardiol, 1987. 59: p. 1271-6.

75. O'Bryne, D.J., S.F. O'Keefe, and R.B. Shireman, *Low-fat, monounsaturate-rich diets reduce susceptibility of low density lipoproteins to peroxidation ex vivo.* Lipids, 1998. **33**(2): p. 149-57.

76. De Stefani, E., *et al., Alpha-linolenic acid and risk of prostate cancer: a case-control study in Uruguay.* Cancer Epidemiol Biomarkers Prev, 2000. **9**(3): p. 335-8.

77. Sugano, M., *Characteristics of fats in Japanese diets and current recommendations.* Lipids, 1996. 31 Suppl: p. S283-6.

78. Pu, Y.S., *Prostate cancer in Taiwan: epidemiology and risk factors.* Int J Androl, 2000. **23**(Suppl 2): p. 34-6.

79. Weisburger, J.H., *Dietary fat and risk of chronic disease: mechanistic insights from experimental studies.* J Am Diet Assoc, 1997. **97**(7 Suppl): p. S16-23.

80. Brawley, O.W. and H. Parnes, *Prostate cancer prevention trials in the USA.* Eur J Cancer, 2000. **36**(10): p. 1312-1315.

81. Nixon, D.W., *Prostate cancer and nutrition.* J S C Med Assoc, 2000. **96**(2): p. 85-6.

82. Masai, M., H. Ito, and T. Kotake, *Effect of dietary intake on urinary oxalate excretion in calcium renal stone formers.* Br J Urol, 1995. **76**(6): p. 692-6.

83. Schwille, P., E. Hanisch, and D. Scholz, *Postprandial hyperoxaluria and intestinal oxalate absorption in idiopathic renal stone disease.* J Urol, 1984. 132: p. 650-5.

84. Trinchierti, A., *et al., The influence of diet on urinary risk factors for stones in healthy subjects and idiopathic reanl calcium stone formers.* Br J Urol, 1991. 67: p. 230-6.

85. Giovannucci, E., *et al., Calcium and fructose intake in relation to risk of prostate cancer.* Cancer Res, 1998. **58**(3): p. 442-7.

86. Curhan, G.C., *et al., Beverage use and risk for kidney stones in women.* Ann Intern Med, 1998. **128**(7): p. 534-40.

87. Schubert, W., *et al.*, *Inhibition of 17 beta-estradiol metabolism by grapefruit juice in ovariectomized women.* Maturitas, 1994. **20**(2-3): p. 155-63.

88. Gupta, M.C., *et al.*, *Effect of grapefruit juice on the pharmacokinetics of theophylline in healthy male volunteers.* Methods Find Exp Clin Pharmacol, 1999. **21**(10): p. 679-82.

89. Grundy, J.S. and R.T. Foster, *The nifedipine gastrointestinal therapeutic system (GITS). Evaluation of pharmaceutical, pharmacokinetic and pharmacological properties.* Clin Pharmacokinet, 1996. **30**(1): p. 28-51.

90. Poortmans, J.R. and O. Dellalieux, *Do regular high protein diets have potential health risks on kidney function in athletes? [In Process Citation].* Int J Sport Nutr Exerc Metab, 2000. **10**(1): p. 28-38.

91. Preuss, H.G., *et al.*, *Effects of diets high in refined carbohydrates on renal ammonium excretion in rats.* Am J Physiol, 1986. **250**(2 Pt 1): p. E156-63.

92. Reyes, A.A. and S. Klahr, *Dietary supplementation of L-arginine ameliorates renal hypertrophy in rats fed a high-protein diet.* Proc Soc Exp Biol Med, 1994. **206**(2): p. 157-61.

93. Michnovicz, J., *Environmental modulation of oestrogen metabolism in humans.* Int Clin Nutr Rev, 1987. 7: p. 169-173.

94. Anderson, K.E., *et al.*, *The influence of dietary protein and carbohydrate on the principal oxidative biotransformations of estradiol in normal subjects.* J Clin Endocrinol Metab, 1984. *59*(1): p. 103-7.

95. Longcope, C., *et al.*, *The effect of a low fat diet on estrogen metabolism.* J Clin Endocrinol Metab, 1987. **64**(6): p. 1246-50.

96. Howie, B.J. and T.D. Shultz, *Dietary and hormonal interrelationships among vegetarian Seventh-Day Adventists and nonvegetarian men.* Am J Clin Nutr, 1985. **42**(1): p. 127-34.

97. Raben, A., *et al.*, *Serum sex hormones and endurance performance after a lacto-ovo vegetarian and a mixed diet.* Med Sci Sports Exerc, 1992. **24**(11): p. 1290-7.

98. Frost, G., *et al.*, *Glycaemic index as a determinant of serum HDL-cholesterol concentration [see comments].* Lancet, 1999. **353**(9158): p. 1045-8.

99. Schurch, M.A., *et al.*, *Protein supplements increase serum insulin-like growth factor-I levels and attenuate proximal femur bone loss in patients with recent hip fracture. A randomized, double-blind, placebo-controlled trial [see comments].* Ann Intern Med, 1998. **128**(10): p. 801-9.

100. Barzel, U.S. and L.K. Massey, *Excess dietary protein can adversely affect bone.* J Nutr, 1998. **128**(6): p. 1051-3.

101.   Sebastian, A., *et al.*, *Improved mineral balance and skeletal metabolism in postmenopausal women treated with potassium bicarbonate [see comments].* N Engl J Med, 1994. **330**(25): p. 1776-81.

102.   Frassetto, L.A., R.C. Morris, Jr., and A. Sebastian, *Effect of age on blood acid-base composition in adult humans: role of age-related renal functional decline.* Am J Physiol, 1996. **271**(6 Pt 2): p. F1114-22.

103.   Nagata, C., *et al.*, *Inverse association of soy product intake with erum androgen and estrogen concentrations in Japanese men.* Nutr Cancer, 2000. **36**(1): p. 14-8.

104.   Klippel, K.F., D.M. Hiltl, and B. Schipp, *A multicentric, placebo-controlled, double-blind clinical trial of beta-sitosterol (phytosterol) for the treatment of benign prostatic hyperplasia.* German BPH-Phyto Study group. Br J Urol, 1997. **80**(3): p.427-32.

105.   Teixeira, S.R., *et al.*, *Effects of feeding 4 levels of soy protein for 3 and 6 wk on blood lipids and apolipoproteins in moderately hypercholesterolemic men.* Am J Clin Nutr, 2000. **71**(5): p. 1077-84.

106.   Anderson, J.W., *et al.*, *Effects of soy protein on renal function and proteinuria in patients with type 2 diabetes [In Process Citation].* Am J Clin Nutr, 1998. **68**(6 Suppl): p. 1347S- 1353S.

107.   Adlercreutz, H., *et al.*, *Inhibition of human aromatase by mammalian lignans and isoflavonoid phytoestrogens.* J Steroid Biochem Mol Biol, 1993. **44**(2): p. 147-53.

108.   Adlercreutz, H., H. Markkanen, and S. Watanabe, *Plasma concentrations of phyto- oestrogens in Japanese men.* Lancet, 1993. **342**(8881): p. 1209-10.

109.   Ajani, U.A., *et al.*, *Alcohol consumption and risk of type 2 diabetes mellitus among US male physicians.* Arch Intern Med, 2000. **160**(7): p. 1025-30.

110.   Molina-Perez, M., *et al.*, *Relative and combined effects of ethanol and protein deficiency on bone histology and mineral metabolism.* Alcohol, 2000. **20**(1): p. 1-8.

111.   Criqui, M.H., *Do known cardiovascular risk factors mediate the effect of alcohol on cardiovascular disease? [In Process Citation].* Novartis Found Symp, 1998. 216: p. 159-67.

112.   Godfroid, I.O., *Eulogy of wine?.* Presse Med, 1997. **26**(40): p. 1971-4.

113.   Tavani, A., *et al.*, *Coffee and tea intake and risk of cancers of the colon and rectum: a study of 3,530 cases and 7,057 controls.* Int J Cancer, 1997. **73**(2): p. 193-7.

114.   Shepard, J.D., *et al.*, *Additive pressor effects of caffeine and stress in male medical students at risk for hypertension [In Process Citation].* Am J Hypertens, 2000. **13**(5 Pt 1): p. 475-81.

115. Lovallo, W.R., *et al.*, *Stress-like adrenocorticotropin responses to caffeine in young healthy men.* Pharmacol Biochem Behav, 1996. **55**(3): p. 365-9.

116. Ezzat, A.R. and Z.M. el-Gohary, *Hormonal and histological effects of chronic caffeine administration on the pituitary-gonadal and pituitary-adrenocortical axes in male rabbits.* Funct Dev Morphol, 1994. **4**(1): p. 45-50.

117. Pizziol, A., *et al.*, *Effects of caffeine on glucose tolerance: a placebo-controlled study.* Eur J Clin Nutr, 1998. **52**(11): p. 846-9.

118. Kleiner, S.M., *Water: an essential but overlooked nutrient.* J Am Diet Assoc, 1999. **99**(2): p. 200-6.

119. Chen, Y.D., *et al.*, *Why do low-fat high-carbohydrate diets accentuate postprandial lipemia in patients with NIDDM?* Diabetes Care, 1995. **18**(1): p. 10-6.

120. Jiang, Y.H., R.B. McGeachin, and C.A. Bailey, *alpha-tocopherol, beta-carotene, and retinol enrichment of chicken eggs.* Poult Sci, 1994. **73**(7): p. 1137-43.

121. Kris-Etherton, P.M., *et al.*, *The role of fatty acid saturation on plasma lipids, lipoproteins, and apolipoproteins: I. Effects of whole food diets high in cocoa butter, olive oil, soybean oil, dairy butter, and milk chocolate on the plasma lipids of young men [see comments].* Metabolism, 1993. **42**(1): p. 121-9.

122. Rein, D., *et al.*, *Cocoa inhibits platelet activation and function.* Am J Clin Nutr, 2000. **72**(1): p. 30-35.

123. Lewis, S.J., *et al.*, *Lower serum oestrogen concentrations associated with faster intestinal transit.* Br J Cancer, 1997. **76**(3): p. 395-400.

124. Giovannucci, E., *Nutritional factors in human cancers.* Adv Exp Med Biol, 1999. 472: p. 29-42.

125. Svetkey, L.P., *et al.*, *Preliminary evidence of linkage of salt sensitivity in black Americans at the beta 2-adrenergic receptor locus.* Hypertension, 1997. **29**(4): p. 918-22.

126. Chan, T.Y., *et al.*, *Urinary dopamine outputs do not rise in healthy Chinese subjects during gradually increasing oral sodium intake over 8 days.* J Auton Pharmacol, 1996. **16**(3): p. 155-9.

127. Iwaoka, T., *et al.*, *The effect of low and high NaCl diets on oral glucose tolerance.* Klin Wochenschr, 1988. **66**(16): p. 724-8.

128. Reinhardt, W., *et al.*, *Effect of small doses of iodine on thyroid function in patients with Hashimoto's thyroiditis residing in an area of mild iodine deficiency [see comments].* Eur J Endocrinol, 1998. **139**(1): p. 23-8.

129.   Konno, N., *et al., Association between dietary iodine intake and prevalence of subclinical hypothyroidism in the coastal regions of Japan.* J Clin Endocrinol Metab, 1994. **78**(2): p. 393-7.

130.   Levi, B. and M.J. Werman, *Long-term fructose consumption accelerates glycation and several age- related variables in male rats.* J Nutr, 1998. **128**(9): p. 1442-9.

131.   Gannon, M.C., *et al., Stimulation of insulin secretion by fructose ingested with protein in people with untreated type 2 diabetes.* Diabetes Care, 1998. **21**(1): p. 16-22.

132.   Okuno, G., *et al., Glucose tolerance, blood lipid, insulin and glucagon concentration after single or continuous administration of aspartame in diabetics.* Diabetes Res Clin Pract, 1986. **2**(1): p. 23-7.

133.   Malaisse, W.J., *et al., Effects of artificial sweeteners on insulin release and cationic fluxes in rat pancreatic islets [In Process Citation].* Cell Signal, 1998. **10**(10): p. 727-33.

134.   Vezina, W.C., *et al., Similarity in gallstone formation from 900 kcal/day diets containing 16 g vs 30 g of daily fat: evidence that fat restriction is not the main culprit of cholelithiasis during rapid weight reduction.* Dig Dis Sci, 1998. **43**(3): p. 554-61.

135.   Guerguen, L., *Interactions lipides-calcium alimentaires et biodisponsibilite du calcium du fromage.* Cah. Nutr. Diet., 1992. **XXVII**(5): p. 1014-7.

136.   Wood, R.J. and J.J. Zheng, *High dietary calcium intakes reduce zinc absorption and balance in humans.* Am J Clin Nutr, 1997. **65**(6): p. 1803-9.

137.   Demling, R.H. and L. DeSanti, *Effect of a hypocaloric diet, increased protein intake and resistance training on lean mass gains and fat mass loss in overweight police officers.* Ann Nutr Metab, 2000. **44**(1): p. 21-9.

138.   Edes, T.E. and J.H. Shah, *Glycemic index and insulin response to a liquid nutritional formula compared with a standard meal.* J Am Coll Nutr, 1998. **17**(1): p. 30-5.

139.   Sharma, R.D., T.C. Raghuram, and N.S. Rao, *Effect of fenugreek seeds on blood glucose and serum lipids in type I diabetes.* Eur J Clin Nutr, 1990. **44**(4): p. 301-6.

140.   Khan, A., *et al., Insulin potentiating factor and chromium content of selected foods and spices.* Biol Trace Elem Res, 1990. **24**(3): p. 183-8.

141.   Wolever, T.M. and J.B. Miller, *Sugars and blood glucose control.* Am J Clin Nutr, 1995. **62**(1 Suppl): p. 212S-221S; discussion 221S-227S.

142. Geleijnse, J.M., *et al.*, *Tea flavonoids may protect against atherosclerosis: the Rotterdam Study.* Arch Intern Med, 1999. **159**(18): p. 2170-4.

143. Engell, D., *et al.*, *Effects of serving size on food intake in children and adults.* Obesity Research, 1995. **3**(Supp 3): p. 3815.

144. Pizzari, T. and T.R. Birkhead, *Female feral fowl eject sperm of subdominant males.* Nature, 2000. **405**(6788): p. 787-9.

145. Ramirez-Torres, M.A., A. Carrera, and M. Zambrana, *[High incidence of hyperestrogenemia and dyslipidemia in a group of infertile men].* Ginecol Obstet Mex, 2000. 68: p. 224-9.

146. Kaiser, F.E., *et al.*, *Impotence and aging: clinical and hormonal factors.* J Am Geriatr Soc, 1988. **36**(6): p. 511-9.

147. Hartoma, R., *Serum testosterone compared with serum zinc in man.* Acta Physiol Scand, 1977. **101**(3): p. 336-41.

148. Netter, A., R. Hartoma, and K. Nahoul, *Effect of zinc administration on plasma testosterone, dihydrotestosterone, and sperm count.* Arch Androl, 1981. **7**(1): p. 69-73.

149. Hunt, C.D., *et al.*, *Effects of dietary zinc depletion on seminal volume and zinc loss, serum testosterone concentrations, and sperm morphology in young men.* Am J Clin Nutr, 1992. **56**(1): p. 148-57.

150. Reyes, A.J., *et al.*, *Diuretics and zinc.* S Afr Med J, 1982. **62**(11): p. 373-5.

151. Mendelson, J.H., N.K. Mello, and J. Ellingboe, *Effects of acute alcohol intake on pituitary-gonadal hormones in normal human males.* J Pharmacol Exp Ther, 1977. **202**(3): p. 676-82.

152. Bertello, P., *et al.*, *Short term ethanol ingestion can affect the testicular response to single-dose human chorionic gonadotropin in normal subjects.* J Endocrinol Invest, 1986. **9**(3): p. 249-52.

153. Kolodny, R.C., *et al.*, *Depression of plasma testosterone levels after chronic intensive marihuana use.* N Engl J Med, 1974. **290**(16): p. 872-4.

154. Kunos, G., *et al.*, *Cardiovascular effects of endocannabinoids— the plot thickens.* Prostaglandins Other Lipid Mediat, 2000. **61**(1-2): p. 71-84.

155. Barrett-Connor, E. and K.T. Khaw, *Cigarette smoking and increased endogenous estrogen levels in men.* Am J Epidemiol, 1987. **126**(2): p. 187-92.

156. Jeremy, J.Y. and D.P. Mikhailidis, *Cigarette smoking and erectile dysfunction.* J R Soc Health, 1998. **118**(3): p. 151-5.

157. Sigurjonsdottir, H., K. Manhem, and S. Wallerstedt, *Liquorice-induced hypertension – a linear dose-response relationship*

[2279]. in Endocrinology Society. 2000. Toronto, Canada.

158. Armanini, D., G. Bonanni, and M. Palermo, *Reduction of serum testosterone in men by licorice [letter].* N Engl J Med, 1999. **341**(15): p. 1158.

159. Melis, M.S., *Effects of chronic administration of Stevia rebaudiana on fertility in rats.* J Ethnopharmacol, 1999. **67**(2): p. 157-61.

160. Bindels, A.J., *et al., The prevalence of subclinical hypothyroidism at different total plasma cholesterol levels in middle aged men and women: a need for case-finding?* Clin Endocrinol (Oxf), 1999. **50**(2): p. 217-20.

161. Velazquez, E.M. and G. Bellabarba Arata, *Effects of thyroid status on pituitary gonadotropin and testicular reserve in men.* Arch Androl, 1997. **38**(1): p. 85-92.

162. Donnelly, P. and C. White, *Testicular dysfunction in men with primary hypothyroidism; reversal of hypogonadotrophic hypogonadism with replacement thyroxine.* Clin Endocrinol (Oxf), 2000. **52**(2): p. 197-201.

163. Wassef, G.N., *Lipoprotein (a) in android obesity and NIDDM: a new member in 'the metabolic syndrome'.* Biomed Pharmacother, 1999. **53**(10): p. 462-5.

164. Wu, S.Z. and X.Z. Weng, *Therapeutic effects of an androgenic preparation on myocardial ischemia and cardiac function in 62 elderly male coronary heart disease patients.* Chin Med J (Engl), 1993.

165. Fushimi, H., *et al., Low testosterone levels in diabetic men and animals: a possible role in testicular impotence.* Diabetes Res Clin Pract, 1989. **6**(4): p. 297-301.

166. Spollett, G.R., *Assessment and management of erectile dysfunction in men with diabetes.* Diabetes Educ, 1999. **25**(1): p. 65-73; quiz 75.

167. el-Rufaie, O.E., *et al., Sexual dysfunction among type II diabetic men: a controlled study.* J Psychosom Res, 1997. **43**(6): p. 605-12.

168. Billups, K. and S. Friedrich. *Assessment of fasting lipid panels and doppler ultrasound testing in men presenting with erectile dysfunction and no other medical problems.* in American Urologic Association. 2000. Atlanta, GA.

169. Pritzker, M. *The penile stress test: a window to the hearts of man?* in American Heart Association. 1999. Atlanta, GA

170. Feldman, H.A., *et al., Erectile dysfunction and coronary risk factors: prospective results from the Massachusetts male aging study.* Prev Med, 2000. **30**(4): p. 328-38.

171. Barry, J.M., B. Blank, and M. Boileau, *Nocturnal penile tumescence monitoring with stamps.* Urology, 1980. **15**(2): p. 171-2.

172. Carroll, J.L., M.H. Baltish, and D.H. Bagley, *The use of PotenTest in the multidisciplinary evaluation of impotence: is it a reliable measure?* Jefferson Sexual Function Center. J Sex Marital Ther, 1990. **16**(3): p. 181-7.

173. Takahashi, Y. and Y. Hirata, *Nocturnal penile tumescence monitoring with stamps in impotent diabetics.* Diabetes Res Clin Pract, 1988. **4**(3): p. 197-201.

174. Saypol, D.C., *et al., Impotence: are the newer diagnostic methods a necessity?* J Urol, 1983. **130**(2): p. 260-2.

175. Katznelson, L., *et al., Using quantitative CT to assess adipose distribution in adult men with acquired hypogonadism.* AJR Am J Roentgenol, 1998. **170**(2): p. 423-7.

176. Seidell, J.C., *et al., Visceral fat accumulation in men is positively associated with insulin, glucose, and C-peptide levels, but negatively with testosterone levels.* Metabolism, 1990. **39**(9): p. 897-901.

177. Mokdad, A., *et al., Diabetic trends in the US: 1990-1998.* Diabetes Care, 2000. **23**(9): p. 1278-1283.

178. Renfro, J. and J.B. Brown, *Understanding and preventing osteoporosis.* Aaohn J, 1998. **46**(4): p. 181-91; quiz 192-3.

179. Finkelstein, J.S., *et al., Osteoporosis in men with idiopathic hypogonadotropic hypogonadism.* Ann Intern Med, 1987. **106**(3): p. 354-61.

180. Kujala, U.M., *et al., Physical activity and osteoporotic hip fracture risk in men.* Arch Intern Med, 2000. **160**(5): p. 705-8.

181. Szule, P., F. Munoz, and B. Claustrat, *Bioavailable estradiol may be an important determinant of osteoporosis in men.* Osteoporos Int, 1999. **11**(suppl 2): p. S151.

182. Wehren, L., *et al., Gender differences in mortality after hip fracture.* Osteoporos Int, 1999. **11**(suppl 2): p. S151-152.

183. Stanley, H.I., *et al., Does hypogonadism contribute to the occurrence of a minimal trauma hip fracture in elderly men? [see comments].* J Am Geriatr Soc, 1991. **39**(8): p. 766-71.

184. Wang, C., *et al., Testosterone replacement therapy improves mood in hypogonadal men—a clinical research center study.* J Clin Endocrinol Metab, 1996. **81**(10): p. 3578-83.

185. Margolese, H.C., *The male menopause and mood: testosterone decline and depression in the aging male—is there a link? [In Process Citation].* J Geriatr Psychiatry Neurol, 2000. **13**(2): p. 93-101.

186. Seidman, S.N. and J.G. Rabkin, *Testosterone replacement therapy for hypogonadal men with SSRI-refractory depression.* J Affect Disord, 1998. **48**(2-3): p. 157-61.

187. Booth, A., D.R. Johnson, and D.A. Granger, *Testosterone and men's health.* J Behav Med, 1999. **22**(1): p. 1-19.

188. Organization, W.H., *Contraceptive efficacy of testosterone-induced azoospermia and oligozoospermia in normal men [published erratum appears in Fertil Steril 1996 Jun;65(6):1267].* Fertil Steril, 1996. **65**(4): p. 821-9.

189. Anderson, F.H., R.M. Francis, and K. Faulkner, *Androgen supplementation in eugonadal men with osteoporosis-effects of 6 months of treatment on bone mineral density and cardiovascular risk factors.* Bone, 1996. **18**(2): p. 171-7.

190. Meikle, A.W., *et al., Pharmacokinetics and metabolism of a permeation-enhanced testosterone transdermal system in hypogonadal men: influence of application site—a clinical research center study.* J Clin Endocrinol Metab, 1996. **81**(5): p. 1832-40.

191. Arver, S., *et al., Long-term efficacy and safety of a permeation-enhanced testosterone transdermal system in hypogonadal men.* Clin Endocrinol (Oxf), 1997. **47**(6): p. 727-37.

192. Meikle, A.W., *et al., Prostate size in hypogonadal men treated with a nonscrotal permeation-enhanced testosterone transdermal system.* Urology, 1997. **49**(2): p. 191-6.

193. Ebling, D.W., *et al., Development of prostate cancer after pituitary dysfunction: a report of 8 patients.* Urology, 1997. **49**(4): p. 564-8.

194. Gustafsson, O., *et al., Dihydrotestosterone and testosterone levels in men screened for prostate cancer: a study of a randomized population.* Br J Urol, 1996. **77**(3): p. 433-40.

195. Kennedy, K.J., T.M. Rains, and N.F. Shay, *Zinc deficiency changes preferred macronutrient intake in subpopulations of Sprague-Dawley outbred rats and reduces hepatic pyruvate kinase gene expression.* J Nutr, 1998. **128**(1): p. 43-9.

196. Suescun, M.O., *et al., Testosterone, dihydrotestosterone, and zinc concentrations in human testis and epididymis.* Arch Androl, 1981. **7**(4): p. 297-303.

197. Verhoef, P., *et al., Arteriosclerosis,* Thrombosis and Vascular Biology. 17, 1997. **5**(989-95).

198. Jacob, R.A., *et al., Moderate folate depletion increases plasma homocysteine and decreases lymphocyte DNA methylation in postmenopausal women.* J Nutr, 1998. **128**(7): p. 1204-12.

199. Marks, J.W., *et al., Nucleation of biliary cholesterol, arachidonate, prostaglandin E2, and glycoproteins in postmenopausal women.* Gastroenterology, 1997. **112**(4): p. 1271-6.

200. Simon, J.A., E.S. Hudes, and W.S. Browner, *Serum ascorbic acid and cardiovascular disease prevalence in U.S. adults.* Epidemiology, 1998. **9**(3): p. 316-21.

201. Simon, J.A., *et al., Ascorbic acid supplement use and the prevalence of gallbladder disease. Heart & Estrogen-Progestin Replacement Study (HERS) Research Group.* J Clin Epidemiol, 1998. **51**(3): p. 257-65.

202. Simon, J.A. and E.S. Hudes, *Serum ascorbic acid and other correlates of gallbladder disease among US adults.* Am J Public Health, 1998. **88**(8): p. 1208-12.

203. Biswas, N.M., *et al., Effect of ascorbic acid on in vitro synthesis of testosterone in rat testis.* Indian J Exp Biol, 1996. **34**(6): p. 612-3.

204. El-Missiry, M.A., *Enhanced testicular antioxidant system by ascorbic acid in alloxan diabetic rats.* Comp Biochem Physiol C Pharmacol Toxicol Endocrinol, 1999. **124**(3): p. 233-7.

205. Kaul, P., *et al., Calculogenic potential of galactose and fructose in relation to urinary excretion of lithogenic substances in vitamin B6 deficient and control rats.* J Am Coll Nutr, 1996. **15**(3): p. 295-302.

206. Graham, I.M., *et al., Plasma homocysteine as a risk factor for vascular disease. The European Concerted Action Project [see comments].* Jama, 1997. **277**(22): p. 1775-81.

207. Boger, R.H., *et al., Dietary L-arginine and alpha-tocopherol reduce vascular oxidative stress and preserve endothelial function in hypercholesterolemic rabbits via different mechanisms [In Process Citation].* Atherosclerosis, 1998. **141**(1): p. 31-43.

208. Brzozowski, T., *et al., Involvement of endogenous cholecystokinin and somatostatin in gastroprotection induced by intraduodenal fat [In Process Citation].* J Clin Gastroenterol, 1998. **27**(Suppl 1): p. S125-37.

209. Reckelhoff, J.F., *et al., Long term dietary supplementation with L-arginine prevents age-related reduction in renal function.* Am J Physiol, 1997. **272**(6 Pt 2): p. R1768-74.

210. Daly, J.M., *et al., Immune and metabolic effects of arginine in the surgical patient.* Ann Surg, 1988. **208**(4): p. 512-23.

211. Giustina, A., *et al., Arginine blocks the inhibitory effect of hydrocortisone on circulating growth hormone levels in patients with acromegaly.* Metabolism, 1993. **42**(5): p. 664-8.

212. Kelly, G.S., *Insulin resistance: lifestyle and nutritional interventions.* Altern Med Rev, 2000. **5**(2): p. 109-32.

213.   Haak, E., *et al.*, *Effects of alpha-lipoic acid on microcirculation in patients with peripheral diabetic neuropathy [In Process Citation].* Exp Clin Endocrinol Diabetes, 2000. **108**(3): p. 168-74.

214.   Kishi, Y., *et al.*, *Alpha-lipoic acid: effect on glucose uptake, sorbitol pathway, and energy metabolism in experimental diabetic neuropathy.* Diabetes, 1999. **48**(10): p. 2045- 51.

215.   Weisburger, J.H., *Mechanisms of action of antioxidants as exemplified in vegetables, tomatoes and tea.* Food Chem Toxicol, 1999. **37**(9-10): p. 943-8.

216.   Palmieri, L., M. Mameli, and G. Ronca, *Effect of resveratrol and some other natural compounds on tyrosine kinase activity and on cytolysis.* Drugs Exp Clin Res, 1999. **25**(2-3): p. 79-85.

217.   Shoskes, D.A., *et al.*, *Quercetin in men with category III chronic prostatitis: a preliminary prospective, double-blind, placebo-controlled trial.* Urology, 1999. **54**(6): p. 960-3.

218.   Terao, J., *Dietary flavonoids as antioxidants in vivo: conjugated metabolites of (-)- epicatechin and quercetin participate in antioxidative defense in blood plasma.* J Med Invest, 1999. **46**(3-4): p. 159-68.

219.   Murkies, A., *Phytoestrogens – what is the current knowledge?* Aust. Fam Physician, 1998. **27**(suppl 1): p. 547-551.

220.   Divi, R.L., H.C. Chang, and D.R. Doerge, *Anti-thyroid isoflavones from soybean: isolation, characterization, and mechanisms of action.* Biochem Pharmacol, 1997. **54**(10): p. 1087-96.

221.   White, L.R., *et al.*, *Brain aging and midlife tofu consumption [see comments].* J Am Coll Nutr, 2000. **19**(2): p. 242-55.

222.   Ishizuki, Y., *et al.*, *The effects on the thyroid gland of soybeans administered experimentally in healthy subjects.* Nippon Naibunpi Gakkai Zasshi, 1991. **67**(5): p. 622-9.

223.   Van Coppenolle, F., *et al.*, *Pharmacological effects of the lipidosterolic extract of Serenoa repens (Permixon) on rat prostate hyperplasia induced by hyperprolactinemia: com-parison with finasteride.* Prostate, 2000. **43**(1): p. 49-58.

224.   Di Silverio, F., *et al.*, *Evidence that Serenoa repens extract displays an antiestrogenic activity in prostatic tissue of benign prostatic hypertrophy patients.* Eur Urol, 1992. **21**(4): p. 309-14.

225.   Wilt, T., *et al.*, *Serenoa repens for benign prostatic hyperplasia.* Cochrane Database Syst Rev, 2000. 2.

226.   Gerber, G.S., *et al.*, *Saw palmetto (Serenoa repens) in men with lower urinary tract symptoms: effects on urodynamic parameters and voiding symptoms.* Urology, 1998. **51**(6): p. 1003-7.

227.   Schoenen, J., J. Jacquy, and M. Lenaerts, *Effectiveness of high-dose riboflavin in migraine prophylaxis. A randomized controlled trial*

[see comments]. Neurology, 1998. **50**(2): p. 466-70.

228. Schoder, H., *et al., Regulation of myocardial blood flow response to mental stress in healthy individuals.* Am J Physiol Heart Circ Physiol, 2000. **278**(2): p. H360-6.

229. Jiang, W., *et al., Mental stress–induced myocardial ischemia and cardiac events.* Jama, 1996. **275**(21): p. 1651-6.

230. Krantz, D.S., *et al., Prognostic value of mental stress testing in coronary artery disease.* Am J Cardiol, 1999. **84**(11): p. 1292-7.

231. Calkins, J.H., *et al., Interleukin-1 inhibits Leydig cell steroidogenesis in primary culture.* Endocrinology, 1988. **123**(3): p. 1605-10.

232. Harenstam, A., T. Theorell, and L. Kaijser, *Coping with anger-provoking situations, psychosocial working conditions, and ECG-detected signs of coronary heart disease.* J Occup Health Psychol, 2000. **5**(1): p. 191-203.

233. Boscarino, J.A. and J. Chang, *Electrocardiogram abnormalities among men with stress-related psychiatric disorders: implications for coronary heart disease and clinical research.* Ann Behav Med, 1999. **21**(3): p. 227-34.

234. al'Absi, M., S. Bongard, and W.R. Lovallo, *Adrenocorticotropin responses to interpersonal stress: effects of overt anger expression style and defensiveness.* Int J Psychophysiol, 2000. **37**(3): p. 257-265.

235. Siegman, A.W., *et al., Antagonistic behavior, dominance, hostility, and coronary heart disease.* Psychosom Med, 2000. **62**(2): p. 248-57.

236. Owada, M., *et al., Risk factors and triggers of sudden death in the working generation: an autopsy proven case-control study.* Tohoku J Exp Med, 1999. **189**(4): p. 245-58.

237. Weidner, G., *Why do men get more heart disease than women? An international perspective.* J Am Coll Health, 2000. **48**(6): p. 291-4.

238. Vrijkotte, T.G., L.J. van Doornen, and E.J. de Geus, *Effects of work stress on ambulatory blood pressure, heart rate, and heart rate variability.* Hypertension, 2000. **35**(4): p. 880-6.

239. Jaffe, A., *et al., Erectile dysfunction in hypertensive subjects. Assessment of potential determinants.* Hypertension, 1996. **28**(5): p. 859-62.

240. Van Cauter, E., *Putative roles of melatonin in glucose regulation [In Process Citation].* Therapie, 1998. **53**(5): p. 467-72.

241. Scheen, A.J. and E. Van Cauter, *The roles of time of day and sleep quality in modulating glucose regulation: clinical implications.*

Horm Res, 1998. **49**(3-4): p. 191-201.

242. Van Cauter, E., R. Leproult, and L. Plat, *Age-related changes in slow wave sleep and REM sleep and relationship with growth hormone and cortisol levels in healthy men.* JAMA, 2000. **284**(7): p. 861-868.

243. Holsboer, F., U. von Bardeleben, and A. Steiger, *Effects of intravenous corticotropin-releasing hormone upon sleep-related growth hormone surge and sleep EEG in man.* Neuroendocrinology, 1988. **48**(1): p. 32-8.

244. Born, J., *et al., Influences of corticotropin-releasing hormone, adrenocorticotropin, and cortisol on sleep in normal man.* J Clin Endocrinol Metab, 1989. **68**(5): p. 904-11.

245. Spiegel, K., R. Leproult, and E. Van Cauter, *Impact of sleep debt on metabolic and endocrine function.* Lancet, 1999. **354**(9188): p. 1435-9.

246. Feychting, M., B. Osterlund, and A. Ahlbom, *Reduced cancer incidence among the blind [see comments].* Epidemiology, 1998. **9**(5): p. 490-4.

247. Erren, T.C. and C. Piekarski, *Does winter darkness in the Artic protect against cancer? The melatonin hypothesis revisited.* Med Hypotheses, 1999. **53**(1): p. 1-5.

248. Gilad, E., H. Matzkin, and N. Zisapel, *Interplay between sex steroids and melatonin in regulation of human benign prostate epithelial cell growth.* J Clin Endocrinol Metab, 1997. **82**(8): p. 2535-41.

249. Lupowitz, Z. and N. Zisapel, *Hormonal interactions in human prostate tumor LNCaP cells.* J Steroid Biochem Mol Biol, 1999. **68**(1-2): p. 83-8.

250. Moretti, R.M., *et al., Antiproliferative action of melatonin on human prostate cancer LNCaP cells.* Oncol Rep, 2000. **7**(2): p. 347-51.

251. Huerta, R., *et al., Symptoms at the menopausal and premenopausal years: their relationship with insulin, glucose, cortisol, FSH, prolactin, obesity and attitudes towards sexuality.* Psychoneuroendocrinology, 1995. **20**(8): p. 851-64.

252. Smith, J.A., *et al., Human nocturnal blood melatonin and liver acetylation status.* J Pineal Res, 1991. **10**(1): p. 14-7.

253. Frank, S.A., *et al., Effects of aging on glucose regulation during wakefulness and sleep.* Am J Physiol, 1995. **269**(6 Pt 1): p. E1006-16.

254. Rosmond, R., *et al., Mental distress, obesity and body fat distribution in middle-aged men.* Obes Res, 1996. **4**(3): p. 245-52.

255. Van Cauter, E., *et al., Sleep, awakenings, and insulin-like growth factor-I modulate the growth hormone (GH) secretory response to*

GH-releasing hormone. J Clin Endocrinol Metab, 1992. **74**(6): p. 1451-9.

256. Schiavi, R.C., *et al., Diabetes, sleep disorders, and male sexual function.* Biol Psychiatry, 1993. **34**(3): p. 171-7.

257. Aboyans, V., *et al., Sleep apnoea syndrome and the extent of atherosclerotic lesions in middle-aged men with myocardial infarction.* Int Angiol, 1999. **18**(1): p. 70-3.

258. Grunstein, R.R., *et al., Impact of obstructive sleep apnea and sleepiness on metabolic and cardiovascular risk factors in the Swedish Obese Subjects (SOS) Study.* Int J Obes Relat Metab Disord, 1995. **19**(6): p. 410-8.

259. Rosmond, R. and P. Bjorntorp, *Psychiatric ill-health of women and its relationship to obesity and body fat distribution.* Obes Res, 1998. **6**(5): p. 338-45.

260. Bray, G.A. and D.A. York, *The MONA LISA hypothesis in the time of leptin.* Recent Prog Horm Res, 1998. 53: p. 95-117.

261. Marucha, P.T., J.K. Kiecolt-Glaser, and M. Favagehi, *Mucosal wound healing is impaired by examination stress.* Psychosom Med, 1998. **60**(3): p. 362-5.

262. Kiecolt-Glaser, J.K., *et al., Slowing of wound healing by psychological stress.* Lancet, 1995. **346**(8984): p. 1194-6.

263. Virgin, C.E., *et al., Glucocorticoids inhibit glucose transport and glutamate uptake in hippocampal astrocytes: implications for glucocorticoid neurotoxicity.* J Neurochem, 1991. **57**(4): p. 1422-8.

264. Kim, J.J. and K.S. Yoon, *Stress: metaplastic effects in the hippocampus [In Process Citation].* Trends Neurosci, 1998. **21**(12): p. 505-9.

265. Magarinos, A.M., J.M. Verdugo, and B.S. McEwen, *Chronic stress alters synaptic terminal structure in hippocampus.* Proc Natl Acad Sci U S A, 1997. **94**(25): p. 14002-8.

266. Goodman, Y., *et al., Estrogens attenuate and corticosterone exacerbates excitotoxicity, oxidative injury, and amyloid beta-peptide toxicity in Neurochem,* 1996. **66**(5): p. 1836-44.

267. Coker, K.H., *Meditation and prostate cancer: integrating a mind/body intervention with traditional therapies.* Semin Urol Oncol, 1999. **17**(2): p. 111-8.

268. Castillo-Richmond, A., *et al., Effects of stress reduction on carotid atherosclerosis in hypertensive African Americans.* Stroke, 2000. **31**(3): p. 568-73.

269. Buxton, O.M., *et al., Acute and delayed effects of exercise on human melatonin secretion.* J Biol Rhythms, 1997. **12**(6): p. 568-74.

270. Bylesjo, E.I., K. Boman, and L. Wetterberg, *Obesity treated with phototherapy: four case studies.* Int J Eat Disord, 1996. **20**(4): p. 443-46.

271. Wood, P.D. and W.L. Haskell, *The effect of exercise on plasma high density lipoproteins.* Lipids, 1979. **14**(4): p. 417-27.

272. Wei, M., *et al., The association between cardiorespiratory fitness and impaired fasting glucose and type 2 diabetes mellitus in men [published erratum appears in Ann Intern Med 1999 Sep 7;131(5):394].* Ann Intern Med, 1999. **130**(2): p. 89-96.

273. Leitzmann, M.F., *et al., The relation of physical activity to risk for symptomatic gallstone disease in men.* Ann Intern Med, 1998. **128**(6): p. 417-25.

274. Buemann, B. and A. Tremblay, *Effects of exercise training on abdominal obesity and related metabolic complications.* Sports Med, 1996. **21**(3): p. 191-212.

275. Chung, W.S., J.H. Sohn, and Y.Y. Park, *Is obesity an underlying factor in erectiledysfunction?* Eur Urol, 1999. **36**(1): p. 68-70.

276. Rantanen, T., *et al., Midlife hand grip strength as a predictor of old age disability.* Jama, 1999. **281**(6): p. 558-60.

277. Herrmann, H.C., *et al., Hemodynamic effects of sildenafil in men with severe coronary artery disease.* N Engl J Med, 2000. **342**(22): p. 1622-6.

278. LaSalle, M., *et al. You don't have to ride in the Tour de France: Erectile dysfunction in 81 consecutive riders.* in American Urologic Association. 2000. Atlanta, Georgia.

279. Crawford, E.D., 3rd, *et al., The effect of bicycle riding on serum prostate specific antigen levels [see comments].* J Urol, 1996. **156**(1): p. 103-5.

280. Nayal, W., *et al. Influences of gym exercises on the penile oxygen pressure.* in American Urological Association. 2000. Atlanta, Georgia.

281. Fries, J.F., *et al., Running and the development of disability with age [see comments].* Ann Intern Med, 1994. **121**(7): p. 502-9.

282. Fred, H.L. and E.A. Natelson, *Grossly bloody urine of runners.* South Med J, 1977. **70**(12): p. 1394-6.

INDEX

non-insulin dependent diabetes
(NIDDM), 17, 21, 37
norepinephrin, 117, 119
Nutrasweet™, 40
nuts
butternut squash with onions and
pecans, **75**
in Gladiator Diet, 47–48, 52
Javelin salad, **65**

O
obesity. *see* overweight and obesity
oils, choosing, 53
olive oil, 24, 26, 44, 53
omentrum, 10–11
onions with skewered shrimp, fennel
and orange, **83**
oranges
with cinnamon, cayenne and
chocolate, **72**
skewered shrimp, fennel and, **83**
ornithine, 110
osteoporosis, 18, 29–30, 33, 101
overweight and obesity
carbohydrate sensitivity
syndrome, 4
erectile dysfunction (ED), 1
hormone imbalance, 91–94
sleep, 119–120
testosterone,
1, 5–7, 19, 31, 92, 94, 99
testosterone replacement therapy
(TRT), 100–101
oxalate, 28, 29

P
palmetto berries, 112
pancreas, 3, 4, 6, 7
pantothenic acid, 114
papain, 111
papaya tea, 49
PCA (proanthocyanoidin), 47
pear in grilled chicken salad, **68**
pecans in butternut squash with onions,
75
Pecos Bill's poblano and tomato salad,
62
penis pushups, 132–133

pepper, cracked, 48
peppers in Pecos Bill's poblano and
tomato salad, **62**
pepsin, 6
phytoestrogens, 33–35, 112
pinto beans in Cowboy Beans, **70**
pita bread
feta and tomato spread, **63**
Greek Adonis chicken salad, **67**
pituitary gland, 15
plate, portion clock image on, 42
polyunsaturated fats, 29
n-6-polyunsaturated oil, 27
Portabella Pizzas, **71**
portion control, 50–51
prayer, 125
proanthocyanoidin (PCA), 47
Proscar, 112
prostate cancer, 27, 105–106
prostate gland and bicycling, 129
prostate-specific antigen (PSA), 129
protein
L-arginine, 110
digestive processing, 20–21
fructose, 40
in Gladiator Diet, 30–31, 46, 52
glucagon levels, 19–20
hormone imbalance and mood, 5
kidney stones, 29
proper consumption of, 41–42
soy-based foods, 34, 35, 46
protein powder in Bodice Ripper
smoothies, **69**
PSA (prostate-specific antigen), 129
pyridoxal-5-phosphate, 109–110
pyridoxine, 109

Q
quercitin, 35, 111

R
rapid eye movement (REM), 120
recumbent bicycling, 129
red snapper en papillote, **84**
refrigerator, cleaning out, 54
REM (rapid eye movement), 120
resveratrol, 35, 47, 111
riboflavin, 114